THE FASTEST
DIET AND
WORKOUT
EVER

LUCY WYNDHAM-READ

THE FASTEST DIET AND WORKOUT EVER

NEW HOLLAND

For my family who have always believed in me and supported me every step of the way and for Mike, my fiancé who was sadly killed many years ago but who has never left my side and is my shining star.

CONTENTS

CHAPTER FOUR

FASTEST WORKOUTS **104**

CHAPTER FIVE

4-MINUTE WORKOUTS **114**

CHAPTER SIX

WALK/RUN EXERCISES

CHAPTER SEVEN

PLAN YOUR WEEK AHEAD

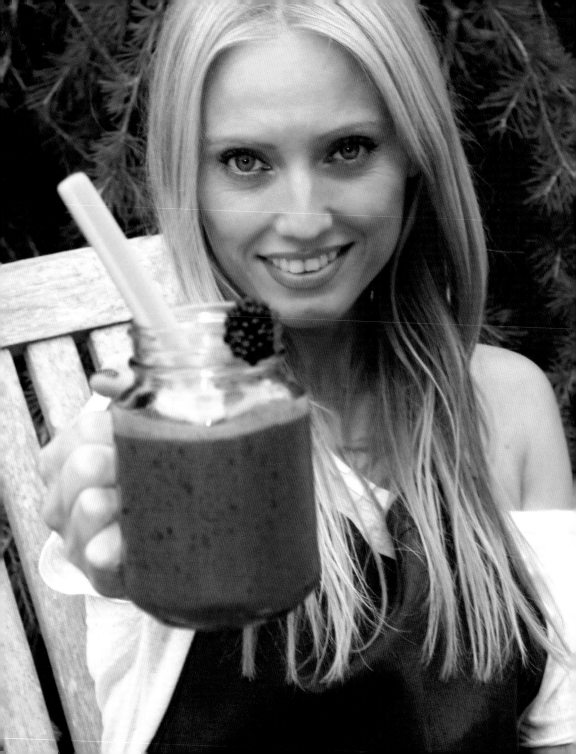

ABOUT LUCY

Lucy Wyndham-Read is a world renowned fitness and weight-loss expert with more than 20 years experience in health, fitness and nutrition.

She began her career in the UK Army and is now the founder of LWR Fitness that specialises in everything to do with health, fitness and leading a healthy lifestyle – regardless of age, gender or different life circumstances. LWR Fitness promotes:

- healthy fitness
- weight loss
- ante- and post-natal health
- body sculpting
- children's health and exercise.

Lucy's passion is to show people how easy exercise and healthy living can be. She has helped thousands of people lose weight and stay in shape. To make it easier than every, Lucy has developed a range of super healthy and anti-aging recipes all of which use clean natural produce so every dish or mouthful is full of goodness and totally delicious.

Lucy is a regular on TV and radio programs giving advice on how to stay fit and healthy appearing on a series on Channel 4 and BBC 1 as a fitness expert. You can also find Lucy's advice in her monthly column in *Feel Good You*. She is a contributor to other magazines and publications including *Glamour*, *Easy Living*, *Marie Claire*, *Look*, *Now*, *Elle*, *Heat*, *OK*, *The Daily Mail*, *The Guardian*, *The Mail on Sunday*, *The Sun* and *Daily Express*.

Lucy is proud to be an Ambassador for HEART UK The Cholesterol Charity, helping to promote awareness and get the word out there about how important fitness is especially for preventing heart disease.

Other charities Lucy has worked with include Macmillan Cancer Support and the Breast Cancer Campaign.

Race For Life is another community project that sees Lucy helping people to get fit and healthy.

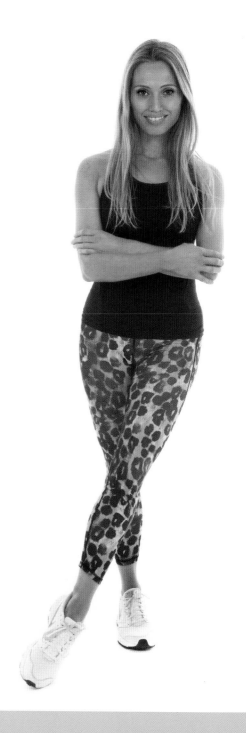

INTRODUCTION

As a fitness and weight loss expert with over 20 years experience, I have seen it all, including crazy diets such as the Tapeworm Diet and the Baby Food Diet, though possibly the craziest idea yet is the Aoqili Diet Soaps that claim to wash away fat. And as for exercise, the gadgets that promise to burn fat and offer miracle weight loss have been equally extreme, from beds you simply lie on and let them do all the toning for you, and fat burning leggings that promise to melt away the fat.

The fact is that weight loss is actually very simple, and more importantly it is easy to maintain for a lifetime. You can do this simply by eating the right foods, in the right quantities and doing the right exercise.

Let me now explain about what's known as the Fast Diet, 5:2 Diet, or as it is sometimes referred to, intermittent dieting. The diet is based on the 5:2 principle. For two days a week, you focus on eating a set amount of calories – 500 for women, 600 for men. For the remaining five days, you simply eat well without a restricted calorie count, but obviously still eating sensible healthy foods. You'll find some delicious recipes and easy-to-make snacks later in the book.

What makes this diet so incredibly successful is that we can all do this. The diet offers you flexibility on the days you choose to do the restricted calorie intake and on the unrestricted days too – and it is sustainable.

This diet is now sweeping the world, but unlike other diets, this one is no passing fad. It is simply a healthy lifestyle that means it is set to stay.

In this book, you'll find out just how many delicious foods you can eat. And honestly, if we eat good healthy foods and in the right quantities, we are spoilt for choice. The foods are nutritious as well as delicious, and when you eat what I refer to as 'fit food', you'll see how easy weight loss can be. You'll want to eat these foods all the time.

Not only will you find a vast variety of recipes, snacks suggestions, meal ideas and tips, but you'll also find out about the other major role in weight loss – fitness. As many diet books overlook the importance of fitness, people struggle to get results. The workouts that go with this fast diet are only four minutes in duration, designed to be quick and get you fast results.

Fitness is a big passion of mine, and I often get emails from people in response to my books, videos and apps saying that, for the first time, they have been enjoying exercise, that these shorter workouts have had amazing results in just a short period of time.

One message I received on Twitter was from a young woman in the United States who said that in just six weeks, following my 4-minute fitness routine which she did four times a week, she had lost more weight than she did when she went to the gym for six months. The point is that these shorter workouts, also known as Fast or HIIT (High Intensity Interval training) get results. In less time you can achieve more.

In this day and age, we are all short of time, so we tend to grab food on the go and forget about exercise. Finding the time to visit the gym for an hour – unthinkable! The good news is you need very little time with my 4-minute workouts to get your body fit.

Let's get going on your new exciting health and fitness, weight-loss journey.

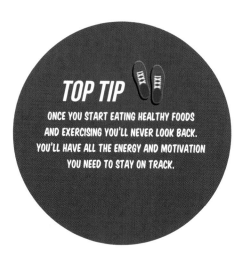

TOP TIP

ONCE YOU START EATING HEALTHY FOODS AND EXERCISING YOU'LL NEVER LOOK BACK. YOU'LL HAVE ALL THE ENERGY AND MOTIVATION YOU NEED TO STAY ON TRACK.

ABOUT THIS BOOK

In Chapter 1 you'll find out how the fastest diet and workout program works and why, what you need and the excellent results you can expect.

Chapter 2 answers some of the frequently asked questions about the diet and workout such as 'can I have a glass of wine with dinner?'

Chapter 3 has the recipes that you can choose from on the two days a week that you will be reducing your calorie count. Surprise, surprise – they are not only low calorie, but delicious and nutritious. You'll find recipes for a week of breakfasts, lunches, dinners and snacks. For your two low-calorie (fasting) days, you can select from the meals or snacks that you fancy.

Each recipe for fasting days includes:

• the time it takes to prepare the recipe

• approximate calorie count
• bonus information about the recipe (if applicable).

Chapter 4 explains how the 4-minute fitness program works and the importance of stretching. It shows how to do stretching exercises for the main muscle groups. Chapter 5 details 10 different 4-minute workouts at various levels of difficulty – but all easy and fast. You'll find illustrations of how to do the 4-minute workouts and information about preparing properly before you exercise that will help prevent injuries and ensure you get the maximum benefit.

Chapter 6 provides information on fat burning, ab toning walking and running exercises that you can add to your exercise program as you wish. The walking and running programs

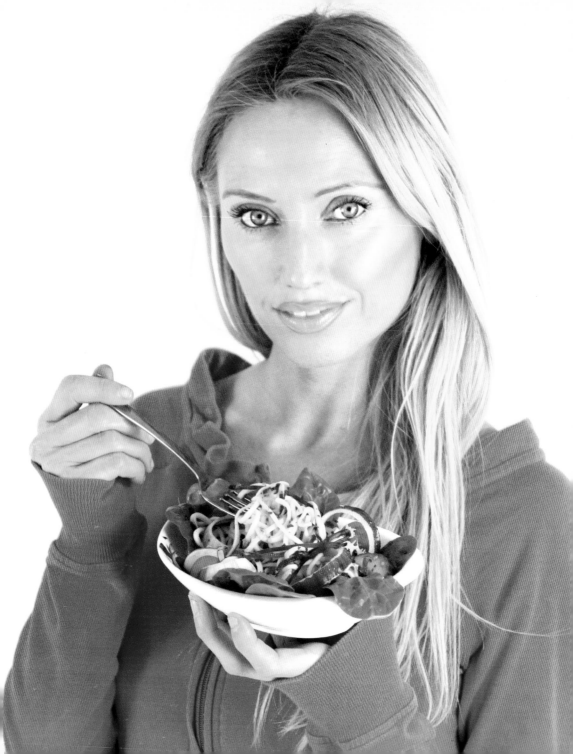

are slightly longer (but still relatively short).

Chapter 7 has a weekly planner that you can use to keep records of your diet and exercise. You'll find 10 top tips for your fasting day and how to stay on target. There is also an example of a weekly diet and workout plan and a template for your weekly plan to photocopy if you wish.

Throughout the book, you'll find top tips and notes that provide additional information to help you get excellent results quickly.

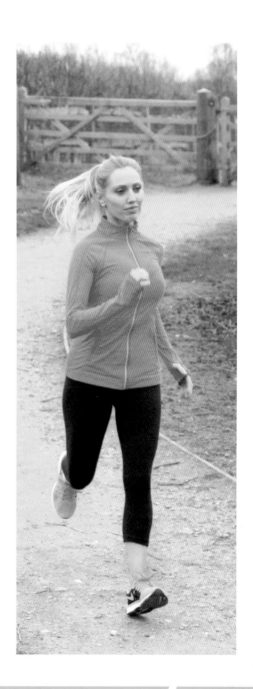

NOTE

FASTING DAYS ARE THE LOW-CALORIE INTAKE DAYS: 500 CALORIES FOR WOMEN, 600 CALORIES FOR MEN. ON NON-FASTING (WORKOUT) DAYS YOUR INTAKE AMOUNTS TO A 'NORMAL' CALORIE COUNT: 2000 CALORIES (WOMEN), 2500 CALORIES (MEN). RECORD THE FOODS AND CALORIES YOU EAT ON YOUR NON-FASTING DAYS TO KEEP AN ACCURATE RECORD OF YOUR FOOD INTAKE OVER A WEEK.

CHAPTER ONE

HOW THE FASTEST DIET/WORKOUT WORKS

The beauty of this diet/workout is that it is so simple. You have two days each week when you simply restrict your calorie intake to 500 calories for women, and 600 calories for men. On the other five days, you eat normally and just make sure you eat good 'fit' foods (which I discuss in more detail later in this book). You don't have to be weighing yourself or religiously counting calories on these days.

Whatever your lifestyle, you can make the diet fit you. Choose your two days for restricting your calories that works for your lifestyle. For example, you may choose Monday and Thursday. If it suits better, you can do two days of low calorie intake, then five consecutive days of normal eating. On these days,

you do the 4-minute workouts at the time of day that suits you.

The great thing about this diet/workout is the flexibility. Throughout the book you'll find lots of tips and ideas on how to stick to this, and more importantly, how to enjoy it.

As for motivation, this will happen quickly. Within a week you will start to notice a difference. By week two, other people will also notice a change, and in week 3, you will feel and look amazing. Do I need say any more?

So, in summary, the Fastest Diet (also known as the 5:2 Diet, the 2-day Diet or intermittent dieting) works on a basis of having two days in any one week to diet when you simply reduce your daily calorie intake on these days.

For the other five days, eat healthily without calorie counting and do the 4-minute (fast) workouts. The result of this is healthy weight loss. It really is that easy.

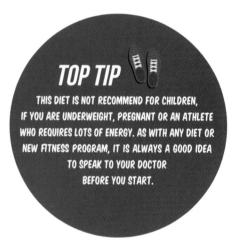

TOP TIP

THIS DIET IS NOT RECOMMEND FOR CHILDREN, IF YOU ARE UNDERWEIGHT, PREGNANT OR AN ATHLETE WHO REQUIRES LOTS OF ENERGY. AS WITH ANY DIET OR NEW FITNESS PROGRAM, IT IS ALWAYS A GOOD IDEA TO SPEAK TO YOUR DOCTOR BEFORE YOU START.

WHAT YOU NEED TO GET STARTED

There is not much you need to start on your new healthy journey, but there are a few things that I would recommend that you think of investing in, and I will explain why.

Before you start, it is important to have at least these five things.

For this you don't need to buy or invest in a whole new workout wardrobe, but I recommend that you have a decent pair of trainers as this will help protect your joints while exercising and make the workout more comfortable. Loose fitting t-shirts and shorts are quite functional or, if colder climates, a tracksuit will suffice.

For women, it is definitely wise to invest in a good sports bra as this again protects you and keeps you feeling comfortable.

A stopwatch is something you will need for your workouts, as they are all timed – and super fast. You don't have to do anymore than the time allocated. Because I have created the workouts with short-interval bursts, a stopwatch will help you stick to the workout times. Many smartphones have a built-in stopwatch app or you can search the app store for a free one.

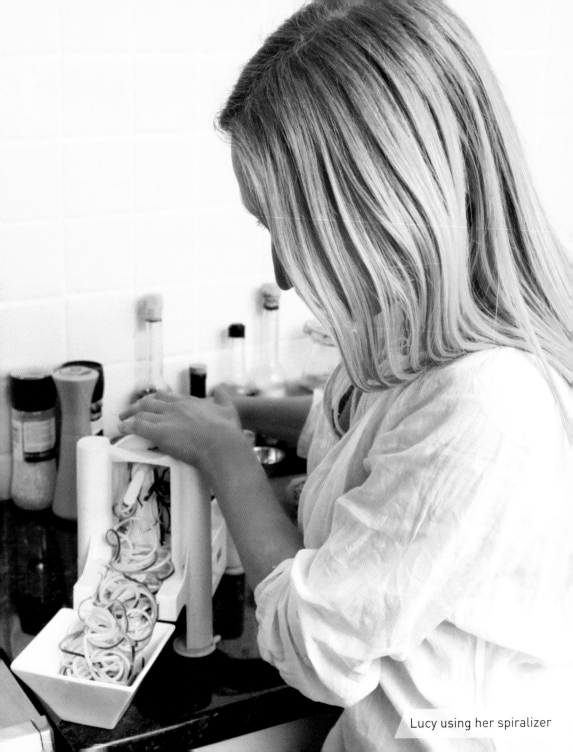

Lucy using her spiralizer

SPIRALIZER

Invest in a spiralizer that is an inexpensive tool that turns fresh veggies into faux-pasta and noodles. They are very popular – everyone from home cooks to restaurant chefs are spiralizing.

For the Fastest Diet, this is great as you can still enjoy all your favourite foods just like Spaghetti Bolognese but with hardly any calories – definitely worth the investment. For example, one medium courgette comes in at 20 calories and it tastes just like spaghetti when it is cooked. I call it my 'courgetti'.

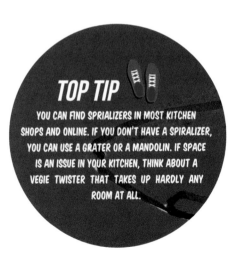

TOP TIP

YOU CAN FIND SPRIALIZERS IN MOST KITCHEN SHOPS AND ONLINE. IF YOU DON'T HAVE A SPIRALIZER, YOU CAN USE A GRATER OR A MANDOLIN. IF SPACE IS AN ISSUE IN YOUR KITCHEN, THINK ABOUT A VEGIE TWISTER THAT TAKES UP HARDLY ANY ROOM AT ALL.

KITCHEN SCALES

It is worth investing a little money in getting some good kitchen weighing scales as these really are going to play a big part on your new healthy lifestyle.

I recommend weighing scales that come with bowls as some of the ingredients we will be weighing will be large in volume so a bowl is ideal.

In the recipes, I have listed weights in the book in both metric and imperial measurements as I am aware that scales vary though most these days can be changed between these two measurement systems.

PEDOMETER

On your non-fasting days, I will recommend certain workouts. However, an additional challenge for you is to accumulate a certain number of steps in a day, as after all it is all about calories in versus calories burned. The more we move, the more we burn. A pedometer will document the number of steps you take. You would be surprised how many steps you take in your daily routine, even just walking around the shops or up and down the stairs. Using this can be a great motivator, as you can set a daily challenge to reach a certain number of steps. You can easily purchase a pedometer – any good sports shop or electronics shop will have them, and there are plenty online.

Every Step Counts: If you are not a big walker, 3,000 a day will start to help improve your fitness. To improve health and prevent weight gain, go for 6,000 steps a day. Anything over 10,000 will help you lose weight and keep you super healthy.

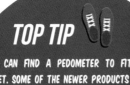

TOP TIP

YOU CAN FIND A PEDOMETER TO FIT YOUR BUDGET. SOME OF THE NEWER PRODUCTS SUCH AS WRISTBANDS CAN TRACK STEPS, DISTANCE, CALORIES BURNED, STEPS CLIMBED SLEEP PATTERNS AND MUCH MORE. SOME SMARTPHONES HAVE FREE APPS WILL MONITOR STEPS TAKEN BUT YOU NEED TO HAVE YOUR PHONE ON YOUR PERSON AT ALL TIMES.

THE RESULTS YOU CAN EXPECT

The combination of eating healthy food and exercising is well known but it's important to reiterate the benefits.

THE BENEFITS OF EATING HEALTHY FOOD

The results from eating healthy foods and exercising are endless and they very quickly start to show. You'll notice a difference in your energy levels, sleep, body shape, fitness and wellbeing. The illustration, 'Food and Health' shows the effects of choosing either healthy or processed foods which have a lot of additives, that is, they can be considered to be 'fake food'.

So every time you eat, refer to the lists showing the benefits of eating fresh or processed as a great motivator to change to healthy, natural food sources. My recipes in Chapter 3 will show you how fresh, clean food not only tastes amazing but will also look after your body.

FOOD AND HEALTH

EATING FRESH FOODS	EATING PROCESSED FOODS
Feeds your body with vitamins and minerals	Provides little or no nutritional value
Helps the body repair itself	Can inhibit the body's ability to heal itself
Helps reduce the risk of disease	Can cause heart disease, diabetes and cancer
Stabilizes blood sugar levels	Causes energy crashes
Prevents weight gain	Causes weight gain
Increase your energy levels	Can make you feel tired and fatigued
Leaves you feeling satisfied and less likely to snack	Leaves you feeling unsatiated and more likely to snack
Helps to slow down the ageing process and gives your skin a natural glow	Can cause excessive bloating and cause discomfort
Helps improve your brain function	Can affect your concentration and bring on depression
Natural food sources, free of additives	Can be harmful because filled with pesticides

THE BENEFITS OF REGULAR EXERCISE

If you have been inactive for a while, it is a good idea to see your doctor before starting your physical activity program. This is particularly the case if:

- you are over 45 years old
- you often faint or have spells of severe dizziness
- moderate physical activity makes you breathless
- you know you are at a higher risk of heart disease
- physical activity causes pain in your chest.
- you are pregnant.

Pre-exercise screening is used to identify people with medical conditions that may put them at a higher risk of experiencing a health problem during physical activity. It is a filter or 'safety net' to help decide if the potential benefits of exercise outweigh the risks for you. Usually, the benefits will far outweigh the risks.

Beginning at a slow pace will allow you to become physically fit without straining your body. Once you are in better shape, you can gradually do more strenuous activity.

If exercise and regular physical activity benefit the body, a sedentary lifestyle does the opposite, increasing the chances of becoming overweight and developing a number of chronic diseases.

If you don't currently exercise and you are not very active during the day, any increase in exercise or physical activity is good for you. Aerobic physical activity – any activity that causes a noticeable increase in your heart rate – is especially beneficial for disease prevention.

The following diagram gives a quick overview of the importance of regular exercise and what happens if you are not exercising.

REGULAR EXERCISE DO'S AND DONT'S

WHEN YOU EXERCISE	WHEN YOU DON'T EXERCISE
You naturally increase the amount of calories your body burns	You body starts to slow down the amount of calories it burns
You reduce body fat levels	Your body stores fat for extra energy
You lose inches all over	Your muscles start to deactivate and become less toned
You increase your heart health	You reduce your blood circulation
You improve your lung capacity	You reduce your energy levels
You increase your feel-good hormones	Your bones become weaker
You keep your muscles toned and active	You can feel depressed and lethargic
You reduce your stress levels	You reduce your concentration levels.
You reduce the risk of high blood pressure	You have less self esteem and confidence
You stimulate the Human Growth Hormone that helps slow down the ageing process	Your body ages faster

CHAPTER TWO

FREQUENTLY ASKED QUESTIONS ANSWERED

How long do I need to be on the diet/ workout before I start seeing results?
You can expect to see dramatic results within the first few days. But instead of jumping on the weighing scales, I suggest you grab a tape measure as this diet and workout is all about losing fat, not muscle. Measure around the narrowest part of your waist and keep a record of this number. You might want to take measurements from other parts of your body too such as hips and top of leg.

Start measuring the day before you begin so you have a record. This will show you how far you have come when you measure yourself at intervals throughout the program – I recommend doing this every couple of weeks. Using the tape measure will show you results as the inches fall away.

Remember, we are all unique so everyone's results will be different but the fact is, if you stick to the diet and do the workouts, you will get those results and you can expect to lose between one and two inches from your waist and in some cases more.

Because I have created this diet with workouts on your non-fasting day, we will not have the problem that 100s of other diets have which can see your weight yo-yoing up and down. This diet is about losing 'fat' and not 'muscle', whereas many other diets can see you losing muscle tissue – which is why when you jump on the scales and get excited about weight loss, if you

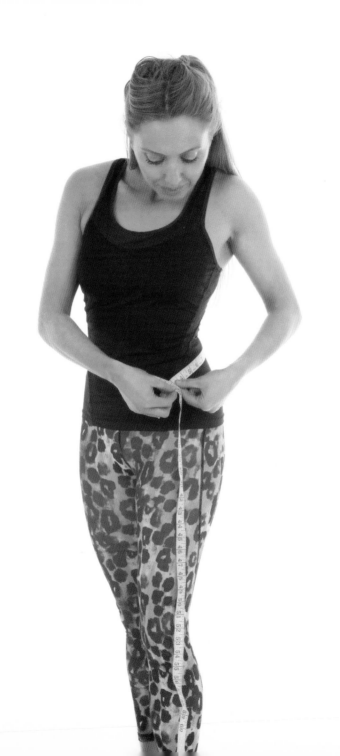

actually measured yourself the inches would be the same. Because muscle tissue is denser (heavier) than fat, weight loss on the scales can mean loss of muscle not fat –the big rolls that we cannot hide.

And the knock-on effect of this is that as you are losing muscle (the less muscle we have, the slower our metabolism). Your body actually starts to slow down its calorie burn, so other diets simply can mean you end up weighing more.

With this diet-workout, we are stripping off the excess body fat and also increasing your muscle tone. The more toned the muscles, the more calories you burn. This is what makes this the 'fastest diet and workout'. It takes a 2-pronged approach. And as the workouts are only 4 minutes, it is so easy to stick to.

For the non-fasting days, can I eat anything I want?

On non-fasting days it is not necessary to count calories, but I would stress to always opt for the healthy version – eating a healthy diet has huge benefits to our wellbeing now and in the long term. To help you to see what would be good to eat on your non-fasting days, have a look at the menu ideas in this book.

You can also see what not to eat in the 'non-healthy' fasting day.

Not only will you benefit from losing fat by following the 'healthy' non-fasting day menu, you'll have more energy.

It's good practice to be aware of how much you eat so simply eat healthy foods and have the right size portions. When you start eating healthy natural

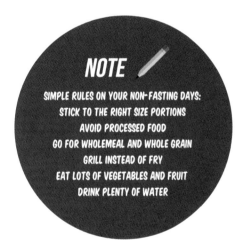

NOTE

SIMPLE RULES ON YOUR NON-FASTING DAYS:
STICK TO THE RIGHT SIZE PORTIONS
AVOID PROCESSED FOOD
GO FOR WHOLEMEAL AND WHOLE GRAIN
GRILL INSTEAD OF FRY
EAT LOTS OF VEGETABLES AND FRUIT
DRINK PLENTY OF WATER

foods, you'll find that you don't crave high fat, high sugar and junk food.

A good way to control this is to think everything we eat either heals us or

NON-FASTING DAY OPTIONS

MEAL	HEALTHY	NON-HEALTHY
Breakfast	Scrambled eggs, grilled mushrooms and grilled bacon with one slice wholemeal toast	Two slices white toast with jam and a bowl of processed cereal (with a high sugar content)
Mid-morning Snack	Latte and a Banana and handful of raisins.	Chocolate bar
Lunch	Grilled chicken breast with wholemeal pasta and sliced avocado and tomato with a balsamic dressing; Low-fat fruit yoghurt	Chicken nuggets and fries; Chocolate milkshake
Mid-afternoon Snack	A couple of crackers with cheese	Crisps and a fizzy drink
Dinner	Homemade Spaghetti Bolognese with a glass of wine.	Pre-brought processed microwave Spaghetti Bolognese. Fizzy drink or several glasses of alcoholic beverage

damages us, so by eating a healthy unprocessed diet, you will be feeding your body with vitamins and minerals and investing in your long-term health as you control your weight.

Of course, we are all allowed the odd bar of chocolate or slice of cake, but just make sure it is once in a blue moon.

On the non-fasting days, is there a 'reasonable calorie count' that will help me to make sure I burn fat and lose inches? What would be appropriate for women and men?

Good question. To get the most out of your non-fasting days, aim to keep your calorie count to around 1700 for women and 2200 for men. But more than anything on your non-fasting days, instead of calorie counting just focus on eating the right sized portions. For further information, find portion guide on my website, lwrfitness.com under the heading, 5:2 diet plan.

I already have a weekly exercise plan that includes aerobic, weights and stretching (yoga/pilates). Should I add the 4-minute workouts and your walk/run exercise routines to my current weekly program or will my program be a substitute for the 4-minute workouts?

I would highly recommend that you still do the 4-minute workouts as this is all part of the plan for the Fastest Diet and Workout Ever. The 4-minute workouts are designed to elevate your metabolic rate for up to 10 hours. At the burn rate of an average of 35 calories an hour, you can burn up to 350 calories (and this is likely to be a lot higher – the harder you train in those 4-minutes the longer is stays elevated).

So definitely still include the 4-minute workouts and keep doing your other exercises. Yoga is excellent exercise for mind and body – a good supplementary exercise program to keep up.

If I want to target a particular area, say muffin top, should I focus on any one particular 4-minute workout or is it best to rotate between them all?

All the 4-minute workouts have the same effect as they quickly burn off excess body fat, but once you have lost the excess body fat and you want to focus on toning a certain part, then you can use these workouts to do just

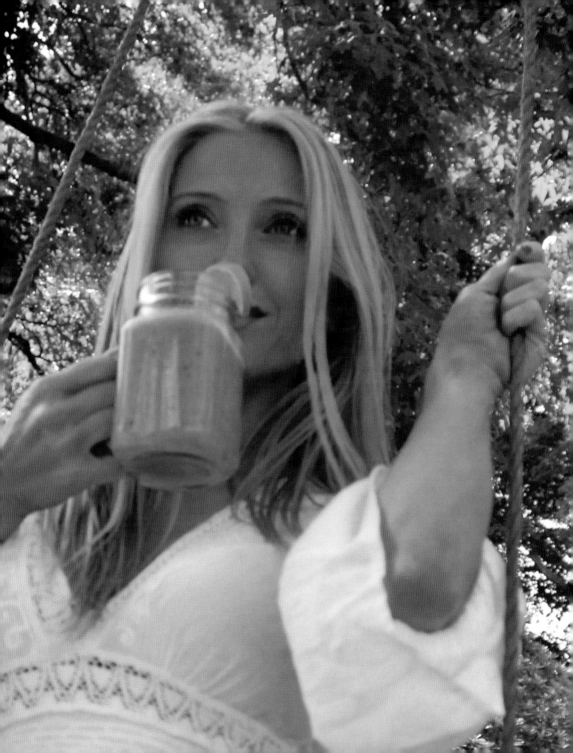

that. Some workouts cross over and tone multiple areas. The following list gives you an idea on what areas each workout targets the most.

FOR THE WAIST, HIPS AND ABS

Wonder Waist Workout

Flat Abs Workout

Skate-it-off Workout

Lower Body Workout

BOTTOM AND LEGS

Squat Jump Workout

Power Jump Workout

No Jump Calorie Burner Workout

Jog-it-off Workout

Skip-it-off Workout

ARMS AND UPPER BODY

Wonder Waist Workout

Skip-it-off Workout

FULL BODY

Fat Burner Workout

Do I make any changes to my program when I get to my goal weight?

Yes, when you reach your goal weight, you can easily maintain it by changing your fasting days from two days a week to just one day a week. On your non-fasting days, for a woman aim to stick to around 2000 calories and for men 2500.

I recommend to do this as you should

never let yourself become underweight. Just as being overweight has negative effects on your health, underweight is also detrimental. Always aim to keep your weight within a healthy range.

How often should I add the longer walk or run workouts?

You could do them once a week. These are in the book to offer variation. They are great to squeeze in during a lunch hour to give you a break from sitting at a desk for long periods of time.

I am in my middle 50s and have tried a lot of diets and exercise to get rid of the extra weight around my waist. How effective is the Fastest Diet and Workout to get rid of midriff fat?

This diet/workout program is highly effective, because it focuses on losing fat not muscle. The 4-minute workouts, unlike other diets, also help to speed up the rate at which your body burns calories. Even while you sleep, you are burning excess calories. When you combine the workouts with the two fasting days, you will see excess body fat drop off fast.

Let's not forget the other benefits

from working out that these 4-minutes give you.

- Increased energy
- Increased fitness
- Reduces stress levels
- Increase your calorie burn
- Sculpts your abs, butt and thighs

I enjoy a drink or two every night. Can I have a glass of wine with dinner on the non-fasting days?

Absolutely! This is a diet that is realistic and life should be enjoyed. So on your non-fasting days enjoy your glass of wine in the evening. Just make sure your glass of wine (or other alcoholic beverage) is accompanied by a super delicious and nutritious home cooked dinner.

Do you have any tips for how to prepare for my fasting day?

Yes, always plan what you are going to be eating so you have ingredients and the food prepared. Make sure if you are using the car on your fasting day that it has enough fuel in it, so you don't have to fill it up and be tempted with all the high-fat snacks at the cashier's counter.

The most important advice, which is really essential, is to make sure you get an early night the night before. This means you wake up feeling fresh and have plenty of energy. Lack of good quality sleep increases a hormone known as 'Ghrelin', the hormone that triggers the feeling of hunger. Lack of sleep increases the level of Ghrelin in abundance. An early night with good quality sleep really will make your fasting day feel so much easier.

How can I find out more?

In the Keep In Touch section at the back of this book, you'll find details of my website and social media channels. Please feel free to contact me if you have any other questions.

The next chapter lists many easy-to-make, nutritious, low-cal recipes for your two 'fasting' days. Complete your first week's plan selecting the recipes you want then shop for the ingredients prior to starting. Add the five workouts for your non-fasting days from the workouts in Chapter 5 to your plan.

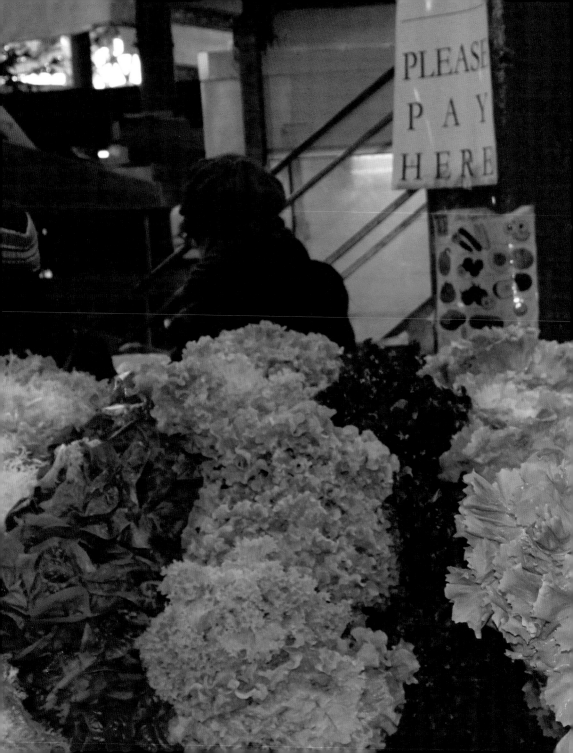

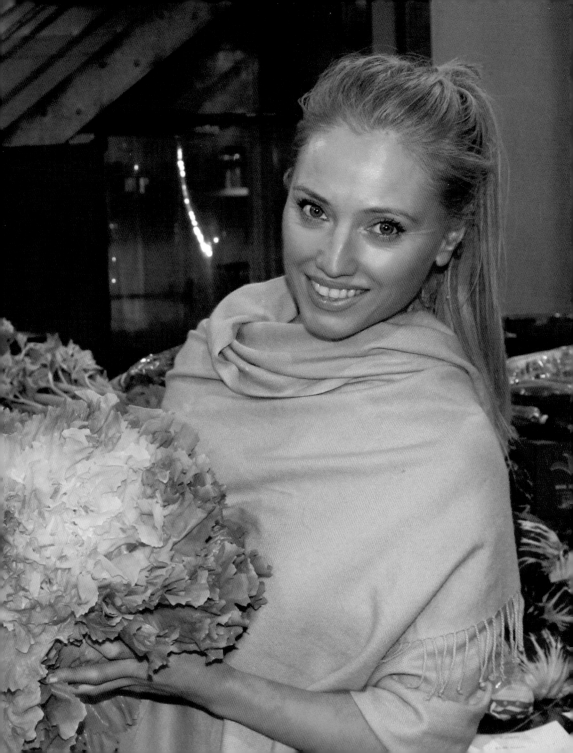

CHAPTER THREE

FASTING-DAY RECIPES

FASTING-DAY BREAKFASTS

Breakfast is one of the most important meals of the day. You'll be amazed at how these tasty the low calorie breakfasts can be – seven recipes, one for each day.

WHY EAT BREAKFAST AT ALL?

Personally speaking, I jump out of bed every morning for breakfast, as it is one of my favourite meals. But many people fall prey to the mistaken notion of skipping breakfast to lose weight, whereas actually this can have the opposite effect. The clue can be found in the word 'breakfast'. If you break down the word, you get 'break' and 'fast' so in fact, you are breaking your overnight fast. While you are sleeping, you obviously have not been eating, and your body has automatically been slowing down to preserve energy and therefore, not using up calories.

Having breakfast breaks that slow pattern – the body and all its systems get back to work full steam. So breakfast is a winner, and even on your fasting days you can still enjoy a tasty early morning treat.

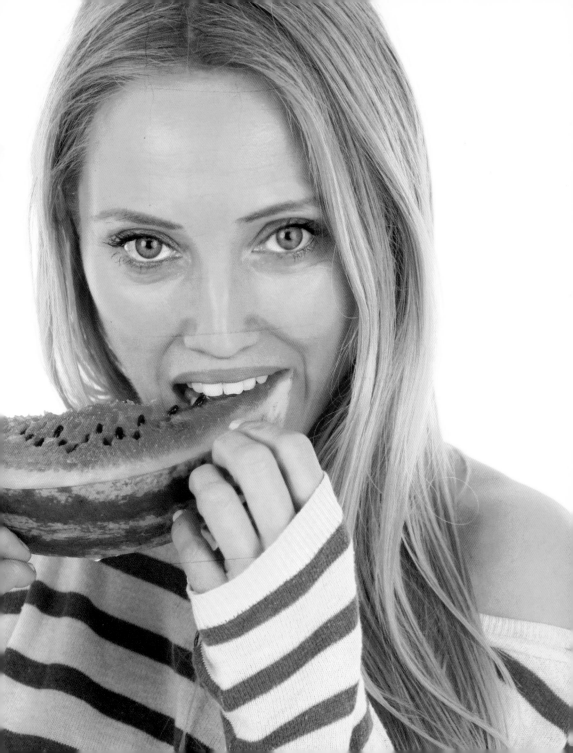

STRAWBERRY & BLUEBERRY CRUNCHY QUARK APPLE POT

Time to make: Under 1 min
Calories: 105

Blueberries are very high in antioxidants making them a great choice for a breakfast.

INGREDIENTS

1 apple
1 teaspoon quark (almost fat-free cream cheese)
3 strawberries
3 blueberries
½ teaspoon almond flakes
½ tablespoon (drizzle) honey

METHOD

1. Simply scoop out a little of the inside of the apple (save the rest of the apple, place in a plastic container and refrigerate for the following day for a snack or smoothie).
2. Add the quark to the apple and top with washed, sliced strawberries and blueberries.
3. Sprinkle with flaked almonds, and finish with a very small drizzle of honey.

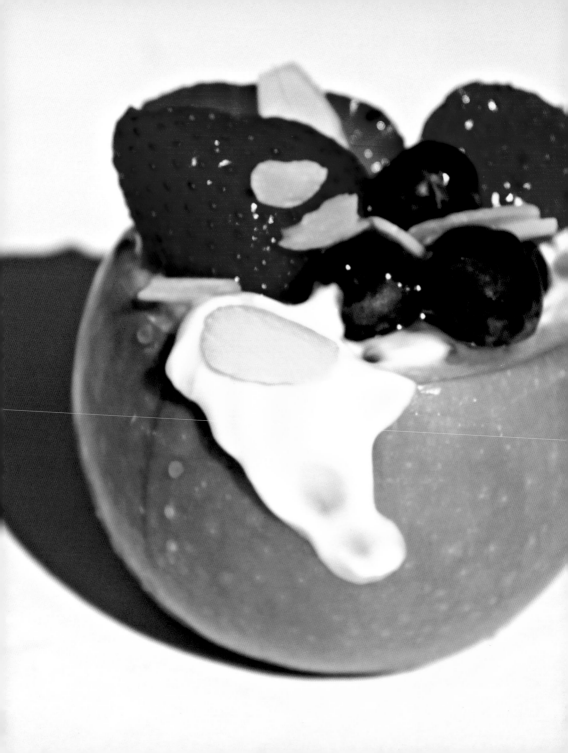

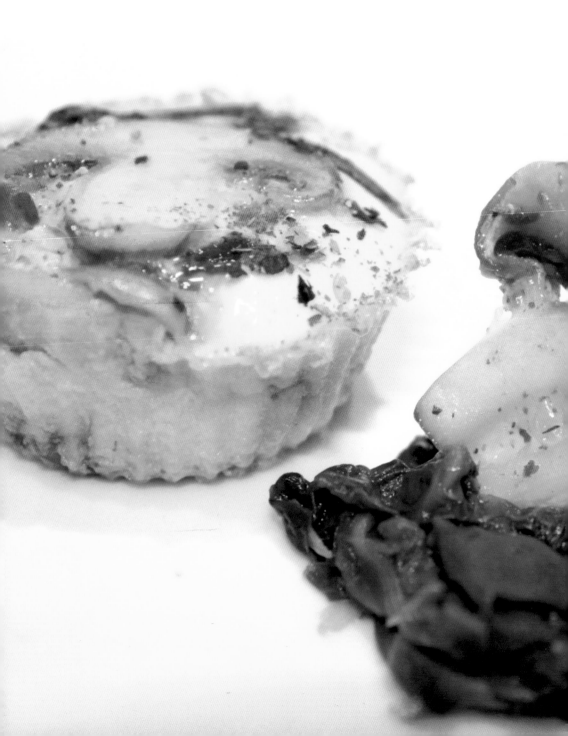

MUSHROOM AND SPINACH CUP CAKE

Time to make: Under 25 min
Calories: 50
Makes approximately 2 cup cakes

BONUS

Nutritionally this breakfast is high in protein, calcium, vitamin A, E, and C, and high in fibre. The chilli helps speed up your metabolism.

NOTE

You can get some super bendy silicone individual cupcake holders that I recommend if you are going to use this recipe a lot.

INGREDIENTS

2 large egg whites
handful of spinach
6 button mushrooms
1 pinch chilli powder
1-cal spray cooking oil (olive oil is a good choice)

METHOD

1. Pre-heat the oven to a moderate heat.
2. Wilt the spinach in boiling water then wash and finely slice the mushrooms.
3. In a non-stick frying pan, add one spray of cooking oil, lightly fry the mushrooms so they are soft, then remove from heat, and once spinach is cooked, remove also.
4. Keep half the spinach and two pieces of mushroom on the side.
5. Break two eggs and decant the egg whites from both into a mixing bowl (You can save the yolks by placing in an airtight container in the refrigerator – they will last for two days). Add the spinach, half the mushrooms yes and the pinch of chilli powder to the egg whites and mix together.
6. Place mixture into cupcake tray. Add two mushroom slices on the top of each cup cake.
7. Place in the middle of the oven at a moderate heat for about 20–25 minutes. Check if cooked by piercing in the middle with a cocktail stick.
8. If it comes out dry, then they are cooked.

GINGER, BLUEBERRY AND PECAN PORRIDGE

Time to make: Under 5 min
Calories: 112
(with maple syrup, 138)

Oats help to stabilise your blood sugar levels and help you feel full for longer.

INGREDIENTS

1½ tablespoons rolled oats
4–6 blueberries
2 crushed pecan nuts
pinch of ginger powder (or ½ teaspoon grated fresh ginger)
water to make porridge
1 teaspoon maple syrup (optional)

METHOD

1. Place the oats in a saucepan with the water (amount of water depends if you like runny or thick porridge).
2. Add a pinch of ginger, simmer and stir constantly until the porridge has thickened to your liking.
3. Remove from pan and pour into a dish. Sprinkle crushed pecan nuts over porridge, and add the blueberries. If you like a sweeter porridge, add maple syrup.

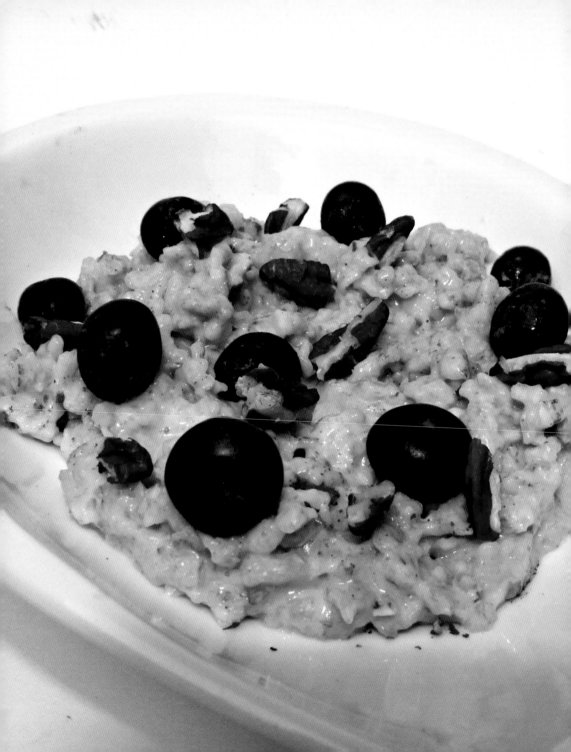

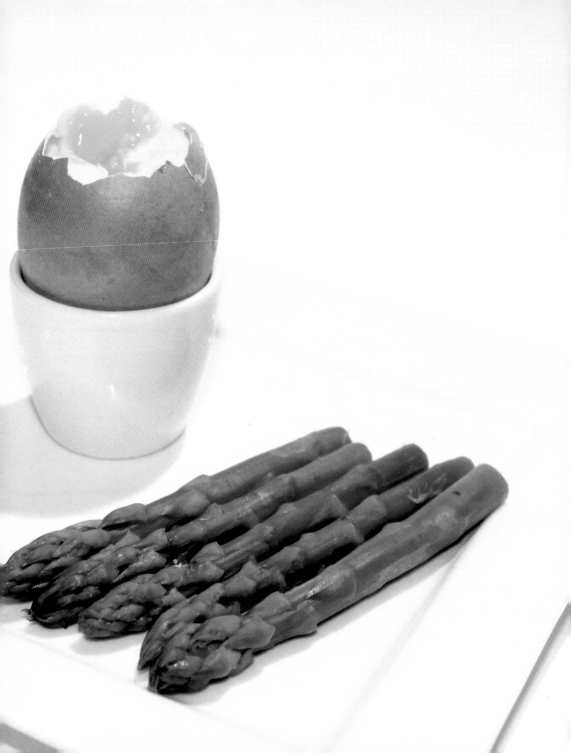

SIMPLE EGG AND GREENS

Time to make: Under 7 min
Calories: 98

BONUS

Asparagus is highly packed with antioxidants and can help to slow the aging process.

NOTE

Cooking times for boiled eggs
3 minutes: The white is set but the yellow is still slightly runny.
4 minutes: The yolk will now be set but should still be runny in the middle.
5 minutes or more: Yolk will be becoming hard

INGREDIENTS

1 medium-sized egg
5 asparagus spears

METHOD

1. Use an egg that has been left out at room temperature for at least half an hour. Add the egg to a small saucepan and fill with enough cold water to cover. Bring the water to the boil. Once boiling, reduce the heat slightly and let the egg simmer. Use a timer to cook the egg to your liking. While your egg is cooking, prepare your asparagus spears. First wash them, and since the base of the asparagus can be tough, it is worth chopping this off.

2. Bring a pan of water to the boil. Add asparagus spears and cook for about 2 – 3 minutes. If you leave them any longer, they can go limp.

3. Once both your egg and asparagus are ready, plate them up and enjoy.

FRUIT SALAD ON TOAST

Time to make: Under 1 minute
Calories: 96

By having wholegrain bread, you can help prevent the body absorbing bad cholesterol.

INGREDIENTS

1 slice wholemeal bread
1 teaspoon low-fat cream cheese
1 large strawberry
1 kiwi fruit
3 blueberries

METHOD

1. Prepare your fruit by cutting into bite-sized pieces and placing in a bowl or on a plate. (If you want to make more fruit for another day, place in an air-tight container and place in refrigerator to use the next day or on your non-fasting day.)
2. Toast the bread and spread with low-fat cream cheese.
3. Top with fruit.

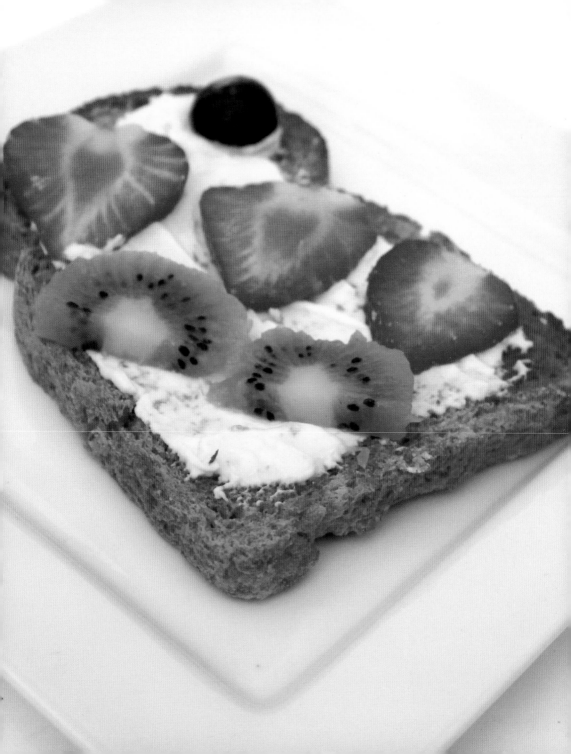

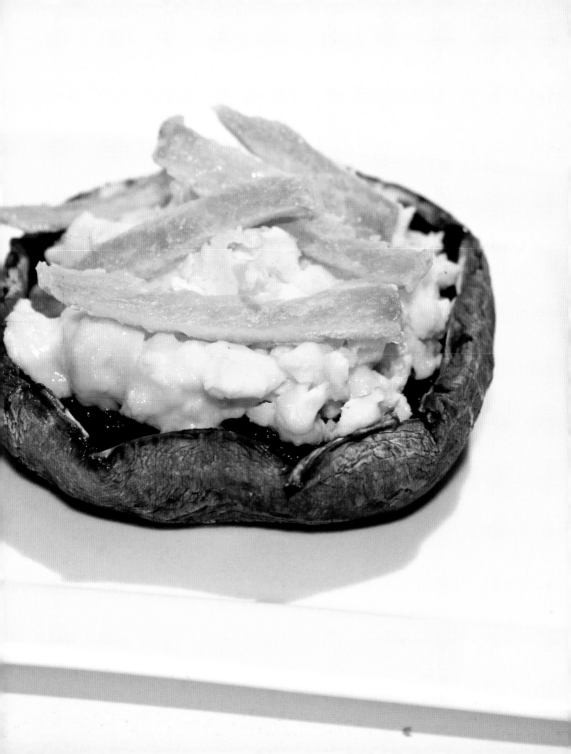

SCRAMBLED EGG AND BACON MUFFIN

Time to make: 25 min
Calories: 181

BONUS

This healthy high-protein breakfast can help to release the hormone Ghrelin that helps to increase the sensation of feeling full for longer.

INGREDIENTS

1 large field mushroom (or 5 button mushrooms)
1 medium-sized egg
1 lean rasher of bacon
½ teaspoon butter

METHOD

1. Preheat the oven to Gas 4/180C (350F).
2. Remove the stalk from the mushroom and wipe away any dirt. Place the mushroom in an ovenproof dish with the cap side down. Add butter to the mushroom. Cook for about 15–20 minutes until tender.
3. To cook your bacon, simply place under the grill. Cook on one side, then turn to cook the other – about 5 minutes or until it is thoroughly cooked.
4. Crack the egg in a bowl and whisk. Add a little seasoning if you wish. Add to a pan on a medium heat and stir constantly. Once cooked, remove from heat.
5. Cut your cooked bacon into strips.
6. Add the egg to the cooked mushroom, and top with the pieces of bacon.

BLACKBERRY CRUMBLE SMOOTHIE

Time to make: Under 1 minute
Calories: 103

BONUS

Blackberries not only add sweetness but also ensure you get plenty of Vitamin K.

INGREDIENTS

75 g low-fat natural yogurt
8–10 blackberries
½ banana
1½ tablespoons rolled oats

METHOD

1. Wash blackberries and peel the banana (any spare banana can simply be put in the refrigerator to use in another smoothie the following day

2. Place all the ingredients into a blender, leaving a few oats and blackberries on the side. Blend all the ingredients, pour into a glass, then top with the remaining oats and blackberries.

3. This smoothie will be thick enough that you can eat it with a spoon, which makes it feel more like a blackberry crumble.

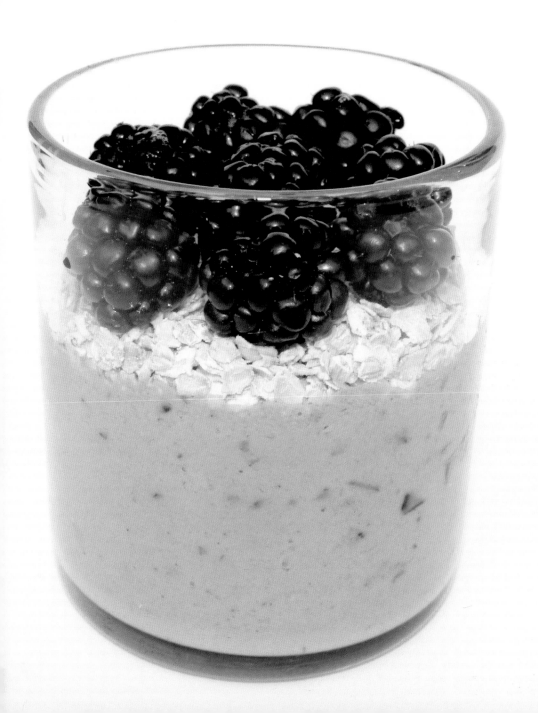

FASTING-DAY LUNCH RECIPES

There's no need to skip lunch on your fasting days, as I have put together seven easy-to-make low-calorie healthy options for you. Using fresh, natural, low-calorie foods will satisfy you, and you really won't feel like you are on a fasting day at all.

When we eat shop-bought lunches and processed foods, these are often laden with hidden sugars and fats that increase the calories. By eating your own prepared food, you are in control of the calories and ingredients. You know what you are eating, thus you know that it is good for you. So feast your eyes over these fasting-day lunches like the Tuna and Red Onion Guilt-Free Pasta that I have even on a non-fasting day as it tastes divine.

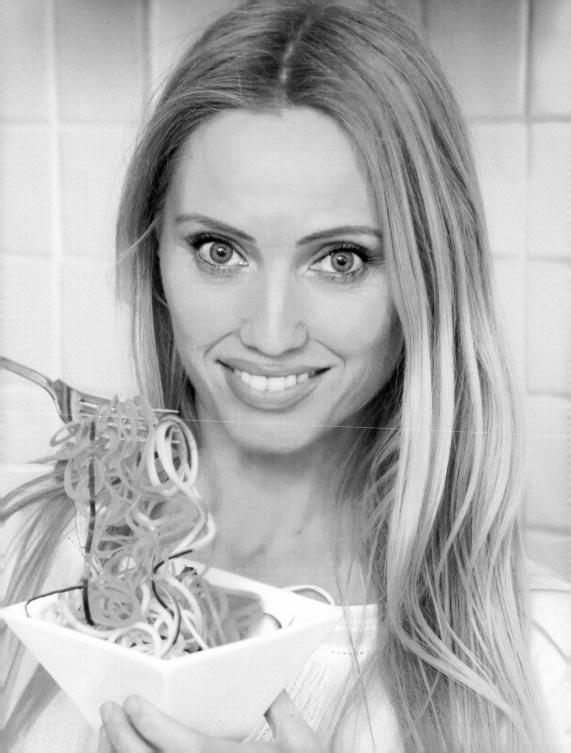

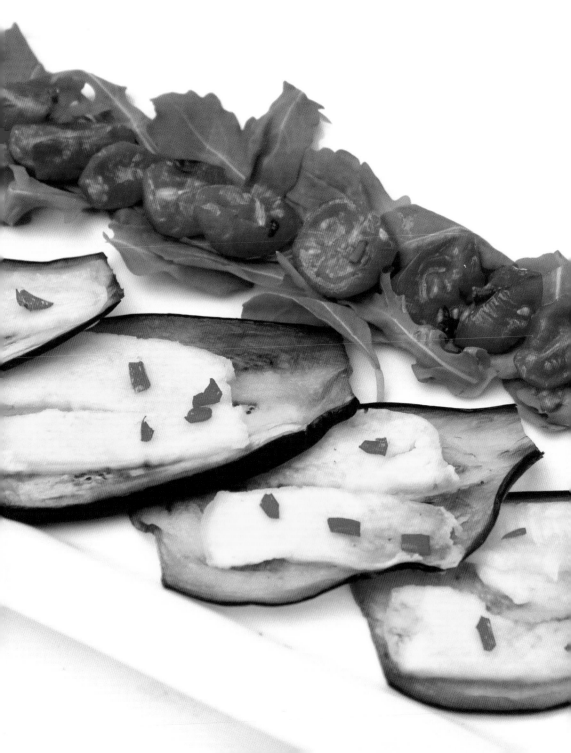

GRILLED AUBERGINE WITH MELTED CHILLI HALOUMI

Time to make: Under 10 min
Calories: 116

BONUS

Aubergines are very low in calories, making them a perfect base for low-calorie dishes. Topping with the chilli flakes helps to increase your calorie burn as they help stimulate your metabolic rate.

INGREDIENTS

125 g (4 oz) aubergine
1½ tablespoons haloumi
6 cherry tomatoes
1-cal spray cooking oil
chilli flakes
handful rocket leaves

METHOD

1. Preheat the oven to a medium heat. Wash and slice your cherry tomatoes and place in a baking tray. Add three sprays of the 1-cal oil. Cook for 10 minutes.

2. Slice the aubergine lengthways, about 6 mm (¼ inch) thick. You will get roughly four slices per aubergine depending on the size. Add one spray of the 1-cal oil.

3. Preheat your grill to a moderate heat and place your aubergine slices under the grill. Grill for approximately 5 minutes turn Add the finely sliced haloumi, sprinkle on the chilli and cook for another 4 minutes or until golden.

4. Serve cooked tomatoes and aubergines on a plate garnished with rocket leaves.

SARDINES ON TOAST

Time to make: Under 1 min
Calories: 124

BONUS
These little fish are full of minerals such as potassium, calcium, iron and phosphorus that help with energy and keeping the body fit and strong.

INGREDIENTS

1 slice wholemeal bread
2 sardines (canned)
1 fresh lemon

METHOD

1. Toast the bread and drain sardines.
2. Place sardines of the toast. Squeeze a little fresh lemon juice over the sardines.

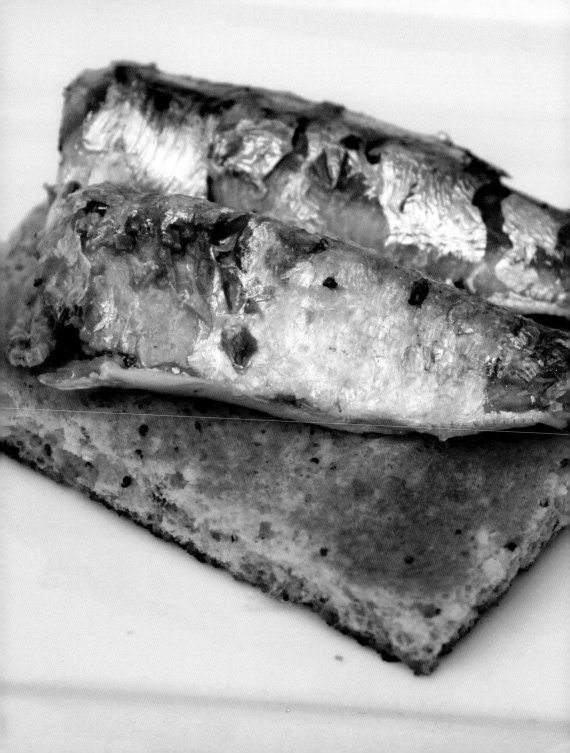

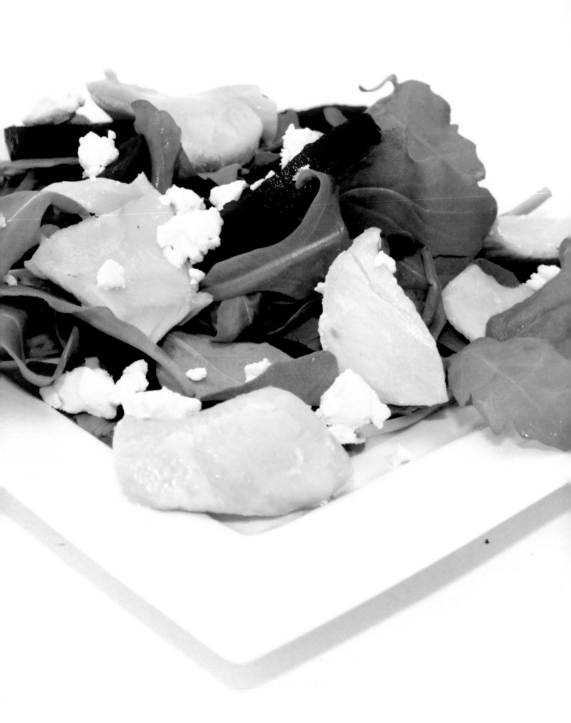

SALMON, BEETROOT AND FETA SALAD

Time to make: Under 2 min
Calories: 141

BONUS

Beetroot can help to lower blood pressure and is very good for your heart.

INGREDIENTS

40 g (1¼ oz) cooked salmon
3½ tablespoons chopped cooked beetroot
1 tablespoon feta cheese
handful rocket leaves

METHOD

1. To prepare, simply wash your rocket leaves and place on a plate with the chopped beetroot.
2. Top with the cooked, flaked salmon and crumbled feta.

MISO AND SPRING VEGETABLE SOUP

Time to make: Under 7 min
Calories: 97

BONUS

Bok choy is a very high source of Vitamin K, which can help make your bones stronger and healthier and delay osteoporosis.

INGREDIENTS

1½ tablespoons miso paste
2 tablespoons baby corn kernels
6 snow peas *(mange toute)*
several leaves bok choy
1 spring onion
1 red chilli
boiling water

METHOD

1. Pour boiling water into a cup. Add the miso paste and stir until dissolved. Transfer to a saucepan over medium heat.
2. Add washed baby corn, bok choy, snow peas, finely chopped spring onion and red chilli. Simmer gently for 4–6 minutes before serving.

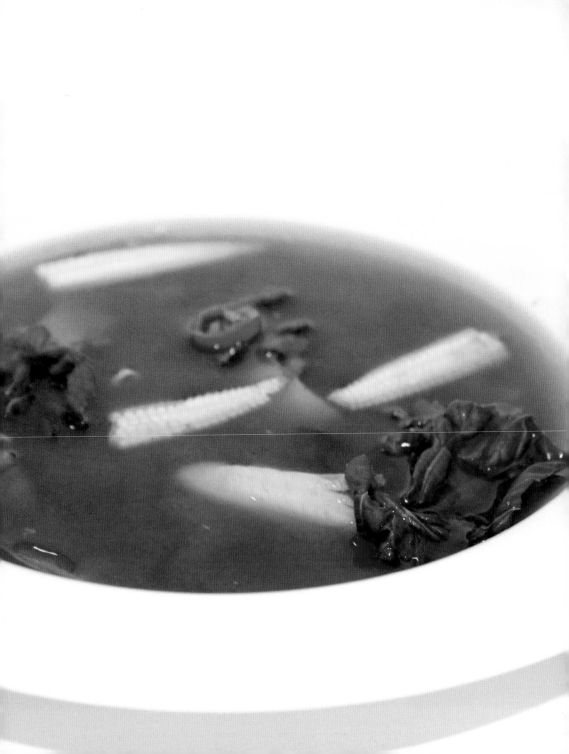

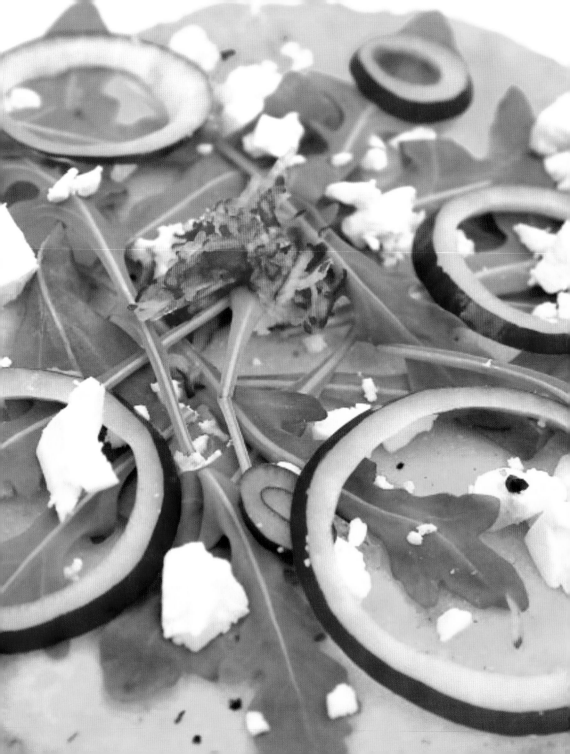

OPEN OMELETTE

Time to make: Under 4 min
Calories: 102

Onions are high in Quercetin and Chromium, which both can be as powerful as Vitamin E to help keep your body in peak condition.

INGREDIENTS

1 medium-sized egg
handful rocket leaves
1 teaspoon feta cheese
1 tablespoon skim milk
¼ red onion, sliced
1-cal spray cooking oil

METHOD

1. Crack the egg into a cup or small bowl and whisk until the yolk is completely mixed. Add a splash of milk.
2. In a frying pan add one spray of a 1-cal oil to a frying pan over medium heat. Pour in the egg mix and allow the egg to cook all the way through.
3. Serve on a plate then top with washed rocket leaves, crumbled feta, and sliced red onion.

LEMON CHICKEN

Time to make: Under 3 min
Calories: 151

BONUS
Having this very high lean protein dish at lunchtime will help to keep you feeling full and your energy levels high all afternoon.

INGREDIENTS
½ cooked chicken breast
2 teaspoon feta cheese
handful rocket leaves
grated lemon zest

METHOD
1. Wash rocket leaves and put them on a plate. Finely crumble the feta over the rocket.
2. Add lemon zest and sprinkle over the salad.
3. Add chicken breast and squeeze a little lemon juice over the top.

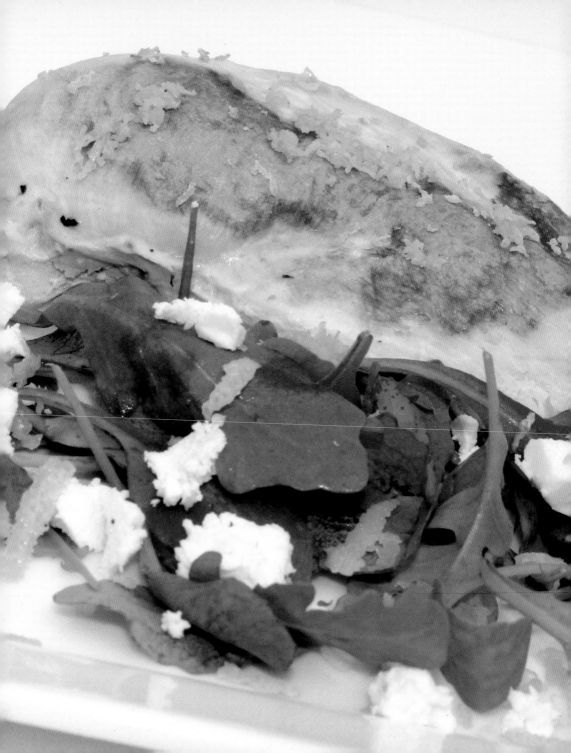

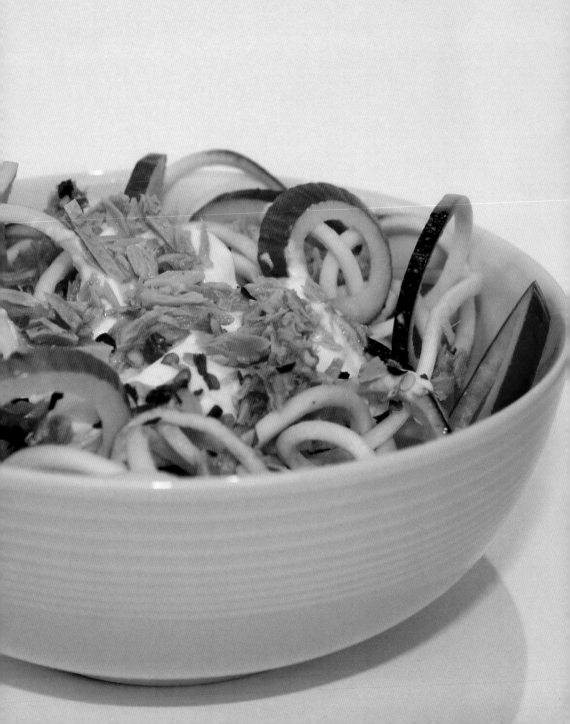

TUNA AND RED ONION GUILT-FREE PASTA

Time to make: Under 2 min
Calories: 145

BONUS

Courgettes are a great alternative to pasta as not only are they super low in calories, they are also very high in the mineral called magnesium which helps to keep our bones strong.

INGREDIENTS

1 medium courgette (zucchini)
⅓ cup tuna (in spring water)
1 tablespoon low-fat natural yogurt
¼ red onion, sliced

METHOD

1. Add the guilt-free pasta to a bowl and top with the drained tuna.
2. Add sliced onion, t a dollop of low-fat natural yogurt and sprinkle on some dried chilli flakes.

TO MAKE GUILT-FREE PASTA

Chop off either end of the courgette (or other vegetable such as carrot, sweet potato or beetroot) and wash. Place in your spiralizer for instant guilt-free pasta ribbons. If you don't have a spiralizer, simply finely grate the vegetables you are using.

You can eat the 'pasta' raw or cook for 1 minute in a microwave oven. If cooking in a saucepan, simply immerse the ribbons in boiling water for no more than a minute.

Another option is to fry your ribbons using 1-cal cooking oil spray. Remember to add each spray to the calorie count for the dish.

FASTING-DAY DINNER RECIPES

Try to eat dinner early and not too late perhaps. If you have any spare calories, you can have a snack after dinner.

Just because you are on a fasting day does not mean you cannot enjoy a nice rewarding dinner, and I would recommend that you have your dinner by 7 pm and avoid eating it any later as we are less active after this time meaning extra calories are more likely to be stored, but you do have a little flexibility with the time as all the dinners are so healthy and low calorie that these don't have a big impact. If you have some extra calories left over from your fasting day budget then your treat yourself to one of the extra snacks.

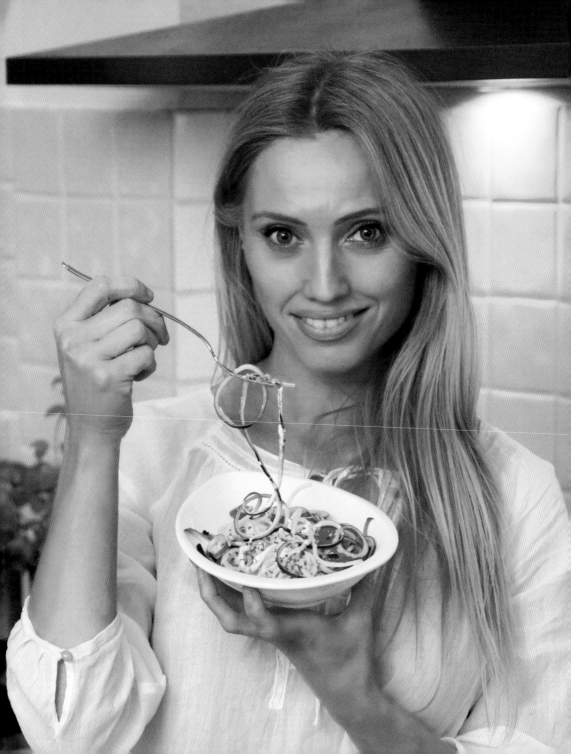

CHILLI CON CARNE

Time to prep: Under 30 min
Calories: 189
(209 with the chilli dip topping)

NOTE

Serve on a bed of 'cauliflower rice'. which tastes similar to rice but with far fewer calories. See recipe (page 101).

INGREDIENTS

⅓ cup extra lean mince
1-cal spray cooking oil
6–8 button mushrooms
¼ red pepper
1 tablespoon red kidney beans
½ teaspoon chilli powder (and other herbs or spices to your taste)
¼ onion
2 tablespoons tomato paste

For chilli dip

½ tablespoons low-fat natural yogurt
1 teaspoon chilli powder

METHOD

1. Finely chop the red pepper, onion and mushrooms. Keep separate.
2. Add 3 sprays of 1-cal cooking oil to a frying pan, add the onions and mince and cook until mince has browned. Add in mushrooms to soften. Remove the mixture from pan and drain off any excess fat. Return to the pan over a medium heat. Add tomato paste, peppers and mushrooms and kidney beans.
3. Add chilli powder and other herbs and spices to your liking. Cover and simmer for 20 minutes.
4. Mix yogurt and chilli powder to make chilli dip.
5. Serve on a bed of 'rice' and top with chilli dip.

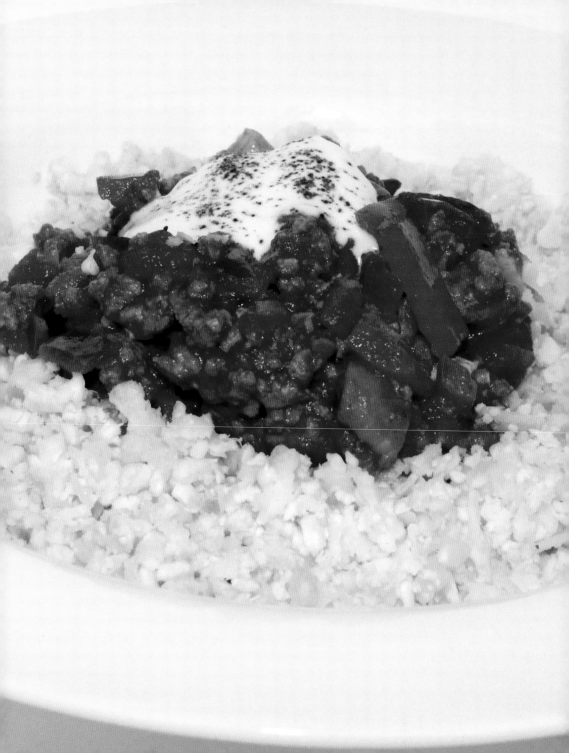

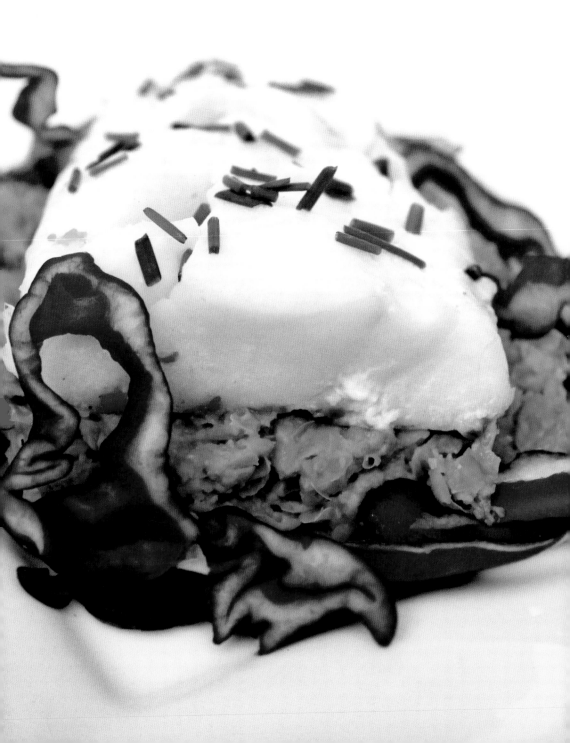

BAKED LEMON AND CHIVE COD ON PEA MASH

Time to prep: 20 min
Calories: 158

BONUS

Peas are cholesterol free, low in fat and sodium and high in protein, which helps to keep you feeling full for longer.

INGREDIENTS

1 cod fillet (120 g/4 oz)
1 teaspoon fresh lemon juice
sprig of chives
2 leaves raw red cabbage (shredded)
4 tablespoons peas (fresh or frozen)
½ tablespoon natural yogurt

METHOD

1. Preheat your oven to a medium heat, 190C (375F). Place a sheet of aluminum foil in a baking dish.
2. Wash the cod fillet and place in the middle of the foil. Pour lemon juice over the fish, fold up the foil so that the cod is sealed tightly.
3. Place in oven. Check on the fish after 10 minutes. Open the foil and if it flakes away easily it is cooked. If not, replace in oven until cooked through. Avoid over-cooking as the fish can become dry and tough.
4. While the fish is cooking, heat some water in saucepan until boiling. Add peas. Once cooked, remove from heat and drain.
5. Place back in saucepan and mash them. Mix in the yogurt.
6. To serve, place the shredded cabbage on the plate. Add the fish and sprinkle with finely-chopped chives.

FILLET STEAK ON CARROT NOODLES WITH BROCCOLI FLORETS

Time to prep: Under 10 min
Calories: 201

BONUS

Broccoli is high in fibre, which aids in digestion, maintains low blood sugar and curbs overeating.

NOTE

A rough guide for cooking steak is: 2 minutes each side for rare, 3 minutes either side for medium, 4 minutes each side for well done.

INGREDIENTS

100 g (3 oz) fillet steak
2 medium carrots
20 g (¾ oz) broccoli
½ teaspoon sesame seeds
1 teaspoon soy sauce (optional)

METHOD

1. Wash and peel the carrot. Spiralize or finely grate and put to one side.
2. Heat some water in saucepan until boiling. Add broccoli and cook for approximately 4 minutes, or until fully cooked. Remove from heat and drain, then break the florets into small pieces.
3. Cook your steak, ideally with a griddle pan as this drains fat, or cook under a grill. Ensure the grill is on a medium to high heat before placing the steak under the grill. Cook to your liking. Allow to rest for 10 minutes. Slice thinly.
4. To serve, place the spiralized or grated carrot on a plate and top with the steak. Add the broccoli florets, and sprinkle with sesame seeds.
5. To add extra flavour, drizzle with soy sauce.

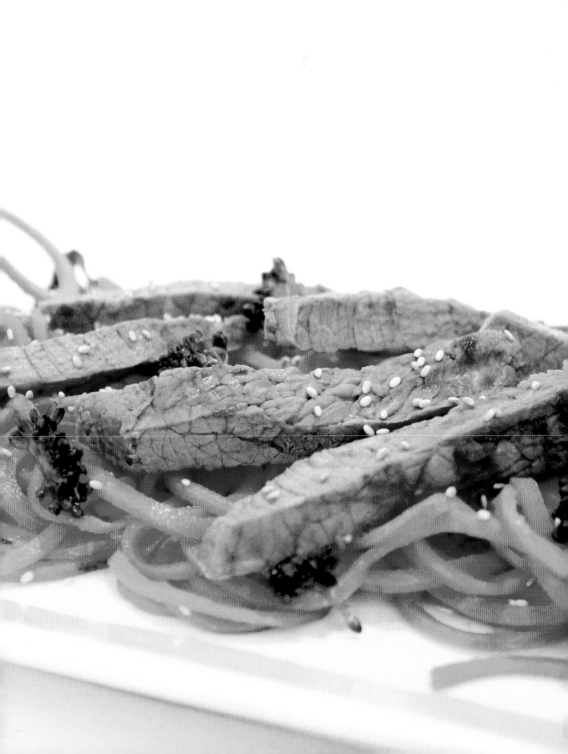

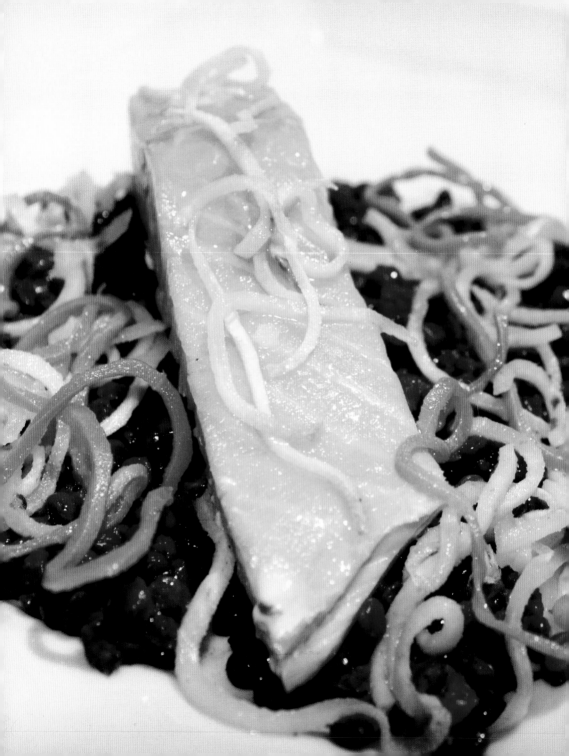

SALMON FILLET WITH CRUNCHY PARSNIP AND CARROT AND PUY LENTILS

Time to prep: Under 20 min
Calories: 255

BONUS

Salmon is very rich in omega-3 fatty acids, which is great for your heart.

NOTE

Cook salmon to your taste: either slightly undercooked in the middle or an opaque colour all the way through. It should flake easily when touched with a fork.

INGREDIENTS

100 g (4 oz) salmon fillet
1 carrot
1 parsnip
2 tablespoons cooked puy lentils (French green lentils)
1-cal spray cooking oil

METHOD

1. Preheat oven to medium hot, 200C (400F).
2. Wash the parsnip and carrot, then spiralize or cut into long thin strips and lay out in an ovenproof dish. Spray with 1-cal cooking oil and place in oven to start cooking.
3. Wrap the salmon fillet in aluminum foil leaving a small opening. Place on ovenproof dish alongside the carrots and parsnips and cook for 16 to 20 minutes. Halfway through cooking, give the carrots and parsnips a stir.
4. Remove from oven and serve the salmon on a plate with cooked puy lentils, adding the crispy carrot and parsnip noodles.

HEALTHY COTTAGE PIE

Time to prep: Under 30 min
Calories: 226

BONUS

Sweet potatoes are high in copper that helps in the production of collagen, which is responsible for keeping muscles healthy and skin taut.

INGREDIENTS

60 g (2 oz) extra lean mince
1 medium sweet potato
2 teaspoons butter beans
¼ red onion, finely chopped
2 tablespoons chopped tomatoes
½ carrot, peeled and chopped
6 green beans (50 g)
handful button mushrooms (10 g/⅓ oz), sliced
1-cal spray cooking oil
coarse black pepper

METHOD

1. Peel and chop sweet potato and cook in boiling water until soft. Drain and mash with a fork. Season with pepper. Set aside.
2. Spray a large shallow pan with 1-cal oil to cover the pan. Add onion and gently fry so the onion is translucent but not brown. Add the mince. Cook for 5 minutes until brown. Add carrots and mushrooms and cook for another 5 minutes.
3. Add tomatoes and beans. Cover the pan and simmer gently for 20 minutes.
4. Add the mince mixture into an ovenproof dish and top with sweet potato mash and cook in a moderately hot 200 C (400F) for 20 minutes. The mash should be crispy on top.
5. Cook green beans in a saucepan of boiling water for 3–5 minutes. Drain and serve cottage pie with the beans.

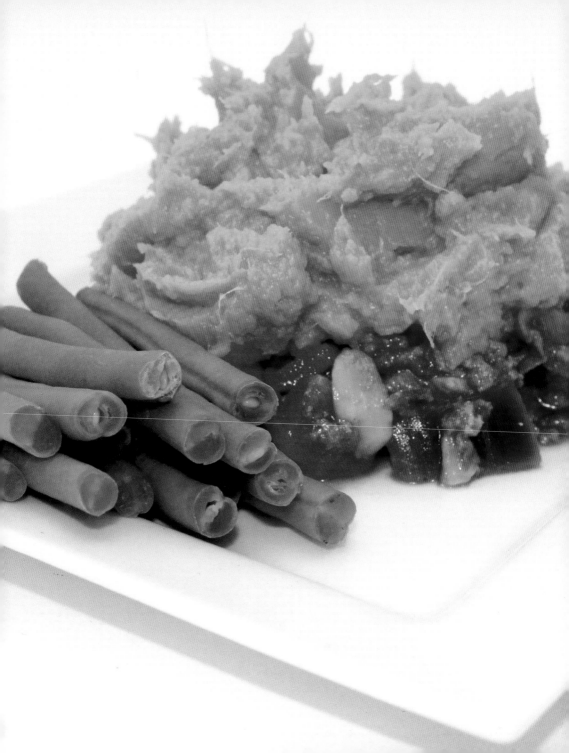

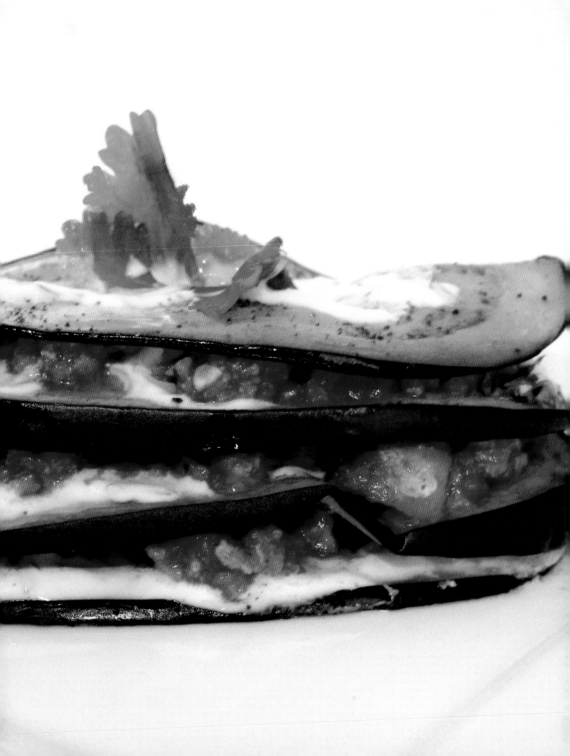

MOUSSAKA

Time to prep: Under 30 min
Calories: 224

BONUS

Aubergine is an excellent source of dietary fibre, and can help protect against type-2 diabetes, and keeps the digestive system regular.

NOTE

If you like a thicker moussaka, add some flour which will thicken the mixture, and stir it in thoroughly (There are 28 calories per tablespoon of flour.) Cornflour mixed with a little cold water is best to use as it blends without forming lumps.

INGREDIENTS

60 g/2 ½ oz low-fat lamb mince
½ aubergine, sliced 6 mm pieces
40 g/1½ oz tinned tomatoes
½ onion, finely chopped
½ tablespoon natural yogurt
1 vegetable stock cube
1-cal spray cooking oil
sprig of parsley

METHOD

1. In a medium to hot pan, spray with oil and lightly cook onion. Add lamb mince (break down the lumps) and cook until brown. Add tomatoes and stock and cook for 20 minutes.
2. While the lamb mince is cooking, spray each slice of aubergine with 1-cal oil. Preheat your grill to a moderate heat and cook aubergine. Cook on each side for about 5 minutes.
3. On a plate, put an aubergine slice, a layer of yogurt, then a layer of mince. Repeat until you have used all the ingredients. Finish with a layer of yogurt.
4. Serve and garnish with a sprig of parsley.

FISH PIE

Time to prep: Under 30 min
Calories: 170

BONUS

Cod is a very high source of protein whilst still being very low in calories and contains lots of Vitamin B.

NOTE

To make toasted breadcrumbs Toast the slice of wholemeal bread. Allow to cook then place in a clean plastic bag. Roll a rolling pin to break it into tiny pieces.

INGREDIENTS

1 cod fillet (100 g/4 oz)
1 medium sweet potato
½ slice wholemeal bread
½ teaspoon butter
lemon juice
sprig of chives

METHOD

1. Preheat the oven to moderate heat 180C (350F).
2. Peel sweet potato and cut into chunks. Add to a saucepan of boiling water. Turn to simmer and cook for about 20 minutes until soft.
3. Place your cod fillet on a baking tray. Mix together butter and a few drops of lemon juice. Smear this mixture on the top of the cod.
4. Place the cod fillet in the middle of the oven and cook for approximately 25 to 30 minutes. When cooked, the fish should flake when touched by a fork.
5. Place the cod in a dish and break the fillet into pieces. Mash the cooked sweet potatoes and place on top of the cod. Add some toasted breadcrumbs to give it a crunchy topping. Sprinkle this over the pie, and finally add some finely chopped chives.

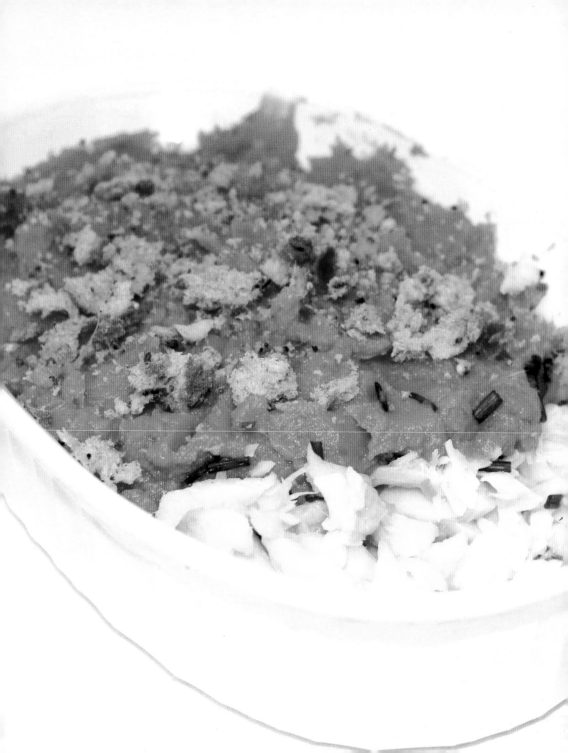

FASTING-DAY SNACK RECIPES

As some of the meals are so low calorie, you will find you have plenty of extra calories from your daily allowance to treat yourself to a tasty snack or smoothie. So if you still have some 'credit' in your calorie allowance, treat yourself to one of these.

These snacks use fresh ingredients, so they will help keep your energy levels high and keep you feeling satisfied.

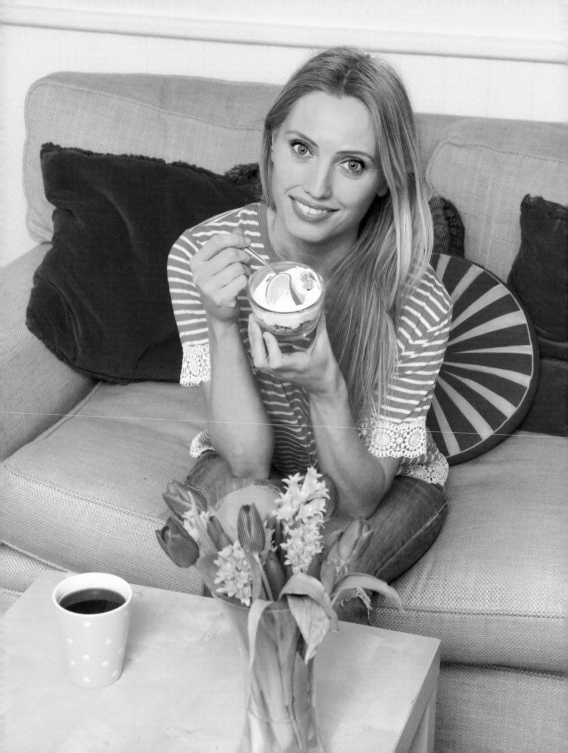

BLACKBERRY AND CELERY CRUSH

Time to prep: Under 1 minute
Calories: 89

BONUS
Celery contains potassium and sodium. If you're not a fan of the taste, don't worry, you can't taste it in this smoothie.

INGREDIENTS
8 blackberries (handful)
8–10 red currants
½ stick celery
6 tablespoons low-fat natural yogurt

METHOD
1. Wash blackberries, red currants and celery. Cut ends off the celery stick. Place ingredients into a blender with the yogurt. Blend until thoroughly mixed.
2. Pour into glass and decorate with celery and blackberries.

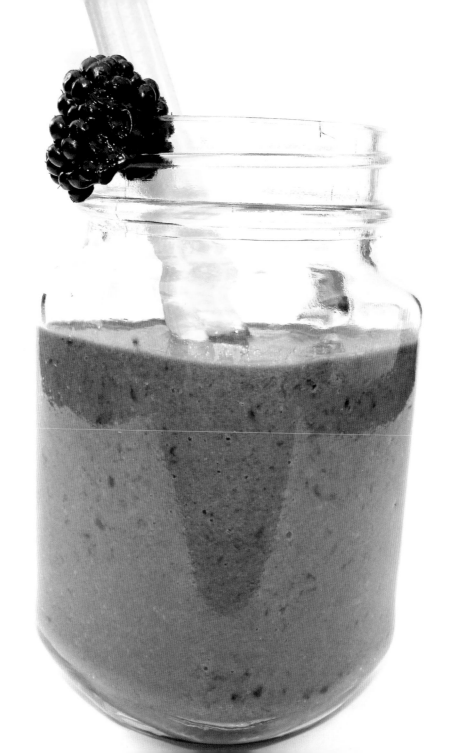

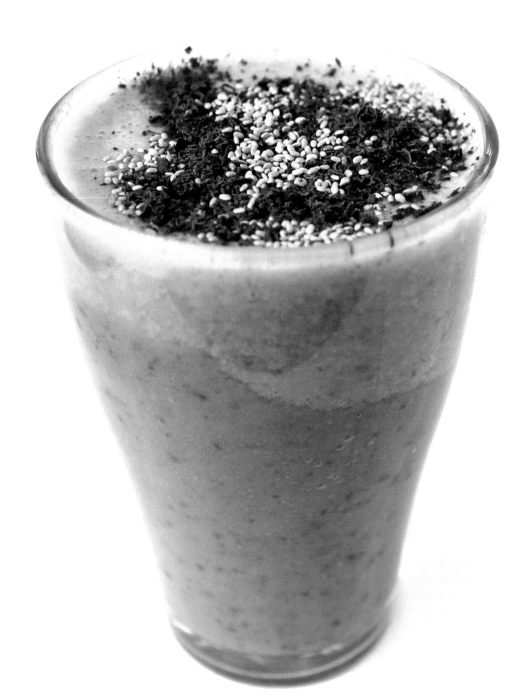

COFFEE AND MOCHA SMOOTHIE

Time to prep: Under 1 minute
Calories: 151

BONUS
Chia seeds are an excellent source of protein, and even though they are quite high in calories (why there's only a teaspoon in this recipe), the health benefits are worth it.

INGREDIENTS
½ lge or 1 sml banana
1 small cup black coffee
125 ml (4 fl oz) almond milk
1 teaspoon chia seeds
10 g/½ oz dark chocolate (finely grated)

METHOD
1. Make a cup of black coffee (instant or espresso). Slightly cool and pour into a blender. Add chopped banana, almond milk, half the dark chocolate and half the chia seeds. Blend until thoroughly mixed.
2. Pour into a glass and top with the remaining chocolate and chia seeds.

FIG AND PUMPKIN SEED SMOOTHIE

Time to prep: Under 1 minute
Calories: 170

Figs are very high in antioxidants, and full of Vitamins A, E and K.

INGREDIENTS

1 sml fresh fig
1½ teaspoon pumpkin seeds
4½ tablespoon low-fat vanilla yogurt
1 teaspoon ground ginger
1 teaspoon honey

METHOD

1. Gently wash the fig and remove the stem. Chop the fig (skin on) into pieces and add to a blender with the yogurt, ginger, honey and half the pumpkin seeds.

2. Blend until thoroughly mixed. Pour into a glass and top with the remaining pumpkin seeds.

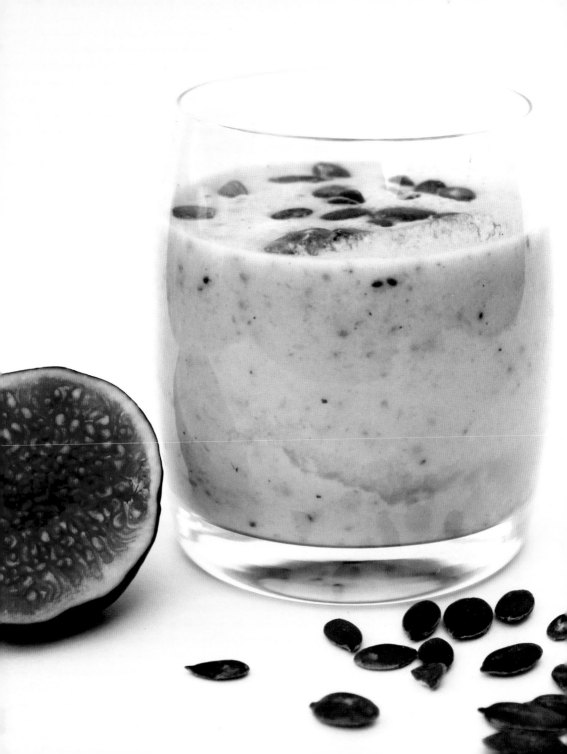

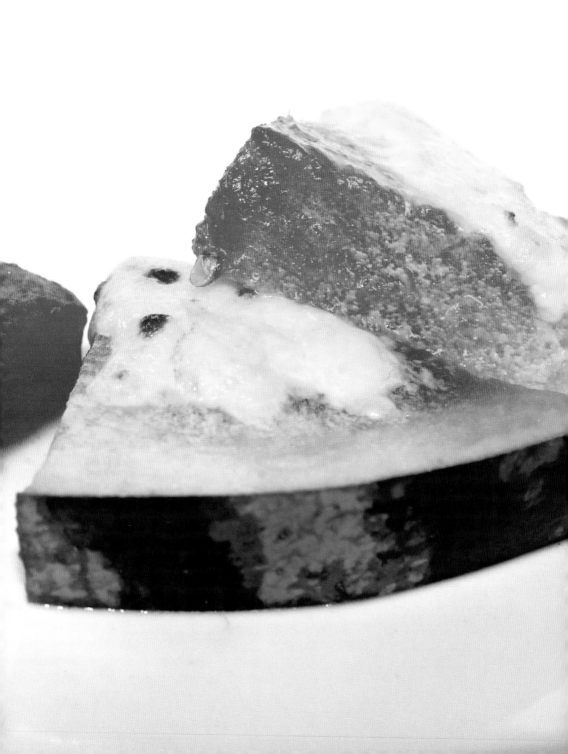

MELON AND MOZZARELLA SLICES

Time to prep: Under 2 min
Calories: 46

BONUS
Heating the watermelon actually brings out its natural sweetness, making this a delicious low-calorie snack, and watermelons are high in Vitamins A, B6 and C.

INGREDIENTS
slice watermelon (60 g/2 oz)
½ tablespoon mozzarella cheese

METHOD
1. Preheat your grill to a medium heat. Cut your wedge of watermelon into 3 small slices, then thinly top with mozzarella over each slice.
2. Place under the grill and cook until the mozzarella starts to go golden. Remove from grill. Allow to cool before eating.

PINK LETTUCE WRAPS

Time to prep: Under 1 minute
Calories: 16

Beetroot is very high in the minerals, potassium and magnesium, as well as Vitamins A, B6 and C.

INGREDIENTS

½ tablespoon low-fat cream cheese
1 tablespoon chopped cooked beetroot
2 lettuce leaves

METHOD

1. Mix the beetroot with the low-fat cream cheese to create a lovely pink mixture.
2. Spoon this mixture into the washed lettuce leaves.

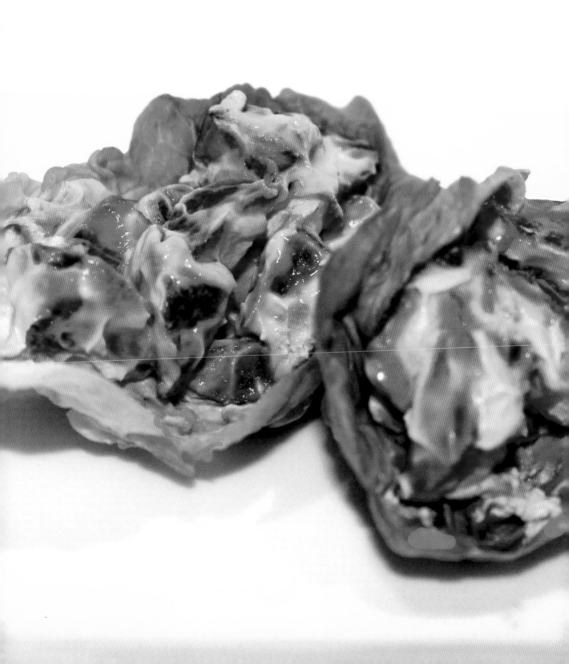

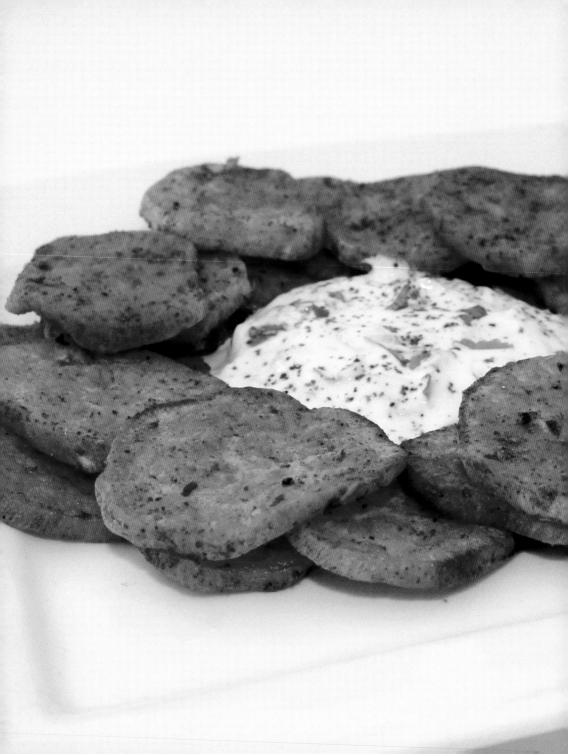

SWEET POTATO CRISPS WITH CORIANDER DIP

Time to prep: Under 25 min
Calories: 54

BONUS
Sweet potato is high in iron, which helps increase your energy levels.

INGREDIENTS

1 medium sweet potato
½ tablespoon low-fat natural yogurt
1 teaspoon coriander
1-cal spray cooking oil
chilli flakes (optional)

METHOD

1. Preheat your oven to moderately hot 200C (400F).
2. Wash and peel sweet potato. Cut into thin slices.
3. Spread out in an ovenproof dish and spray with 1-cal oil. Sprinkle with coriander and chilli if you prefer. Cook for 20 to 25 minutes, or until golden, turning halfway through.
4. To make coriander dip, wash the coriander and tear it into tiny pieces. Mix into yogurt. Serve chips on a platter with a bowl of the dip.

LIME CHEESECAKE

Time to prep: Under 10 min
Calories: 90

Oatcakes are a very low
GI food, which means they
help to stabilize your blood
sugars and keep energy
levels high.

NOTE
Oatcakes – plain biscuits
made with rough oats,
water and salt. Substitute
with digestive or other
plain biscuits.

INGREDIENTS
10 g (½ oz) oatcakes
1½ tablespoon low-fat cream cheese
1 teaspoon honey
zest and juice of a lime

METHOD
1. Place the oatcake in a small plastic bag on a chopping board and break into small pieces using a rolling pin.
2. Put the pieces in the bottom of a small dish.
3. In a bowl, mix the cream cheese with some freshly-squeezed lime juice. Add this mixture to the top of the crushed oatcake.
4. Decorate with a little lime zest and honey.

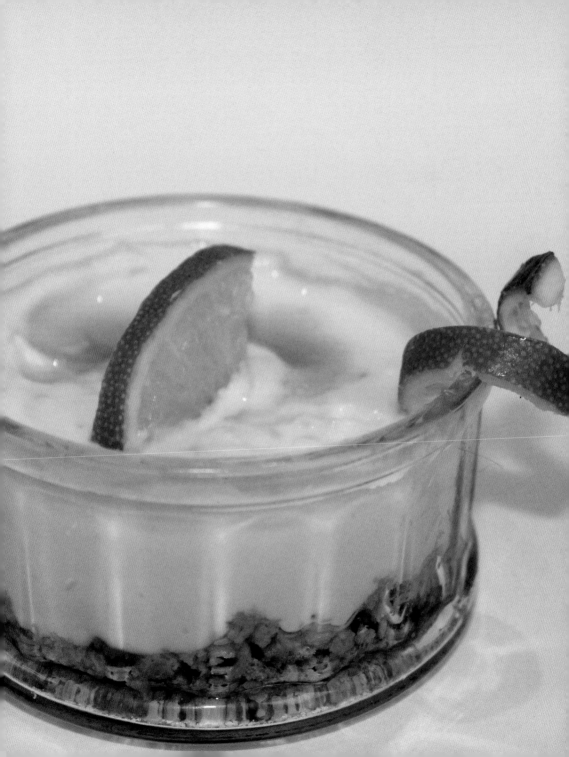

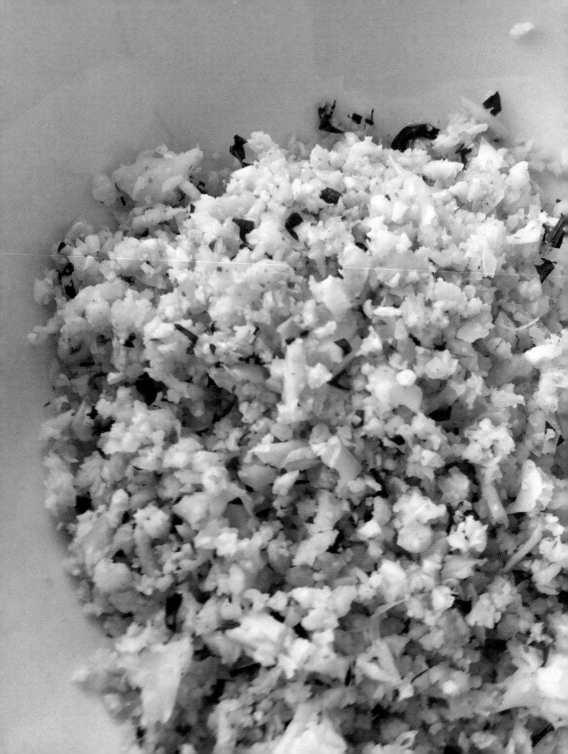

CAULIFLOWER RICE

Time to prep: Under 10 min
Calories: 15

BONUS

Cauliflower is a good source of Vitamin C and Manganese, a mineral that plays an important role in keeping skin healthy.

NOTE

Serve with Chilli Con Carne (page 70). Make a large batch and freeze so it is ready to use for other meals.

INGREDIENTS

1/4 medium cauliflower (about 2 cups of florets)
1 tbs finely chopped parsley

METHOD

1. Wash the cauliflower thoroughly and remove the stalk and leaves.
2. Cut the cauliflower into pieces then cut the florets off the core.
3. Grate the florets finely or place the florets in a blender. The florets should now resemble rice.
4. Heat the 'rice' in a microwave-safe bowl for 10–20 seconds.

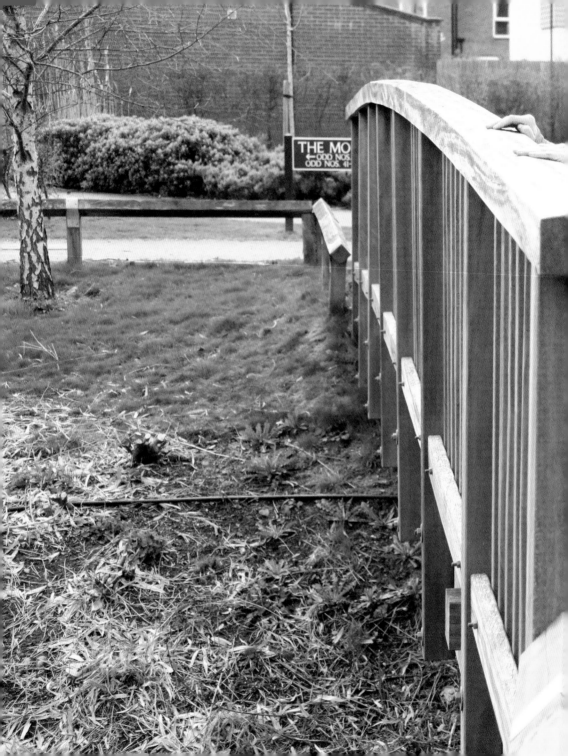

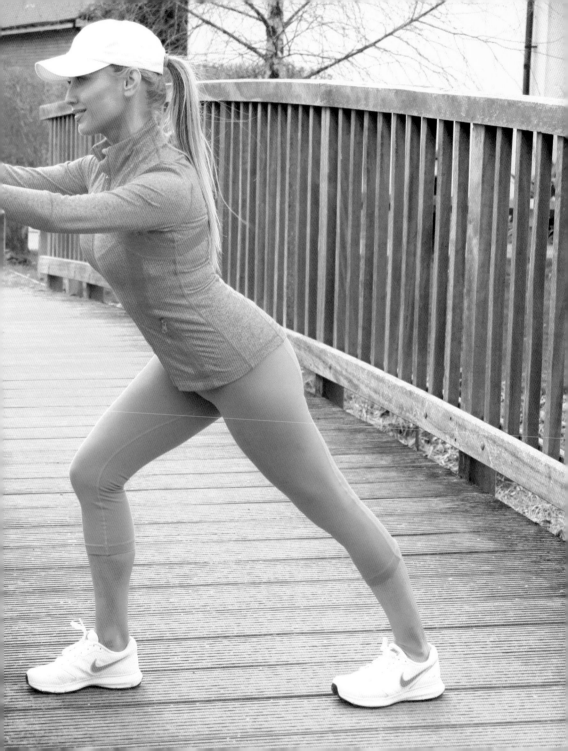

CHAPTER FOUR

FASTEST WORKOUTS

ABOUT 4-MINUTE FITNESS

Your non-fasting days are the days when you will be working on your fitness. This book has over 10 different 4-minute workouts that you can choose from. The benefit is that you will never become bored, as you will have a workout to suit the mood you are in, or your location.

You may wish to keep a record of the specific routine for each non-fasting day on the weekly schedule at the back of the book. This is a great way of really committing; you are more likely to stick to the program if you have written it down.

One of the benefits of 4-Minute Fitness, also known as HIIT (High-Intensity Interval Training) is that the workouts are short. More importantly, you'll see amazing results in a short period of time.

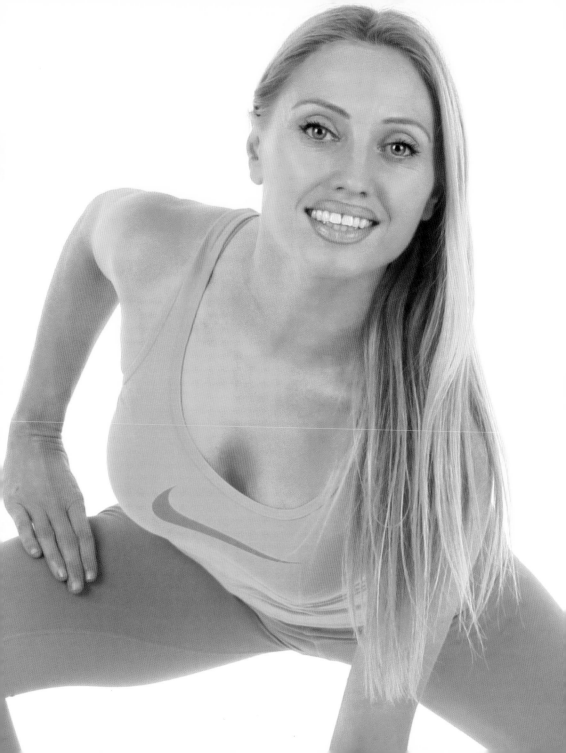

WHY IT WORKS

When we exercise at a high intensity (in other words push ourselves very hard for short bursts of time), we have what's known as an EPOC effect (Excessive Post Oxygen Consumption). This means that after you have finished your workout, your body will be burning calories at an elevated rate for up to 10 hours, at approximately an extra 35 calories per hour, or 350 calories over the 10 hours. This is where these 4-minute workouts are amazing – long after you have finished working out, you're still burning calories.

This is why intensity is the most important part of a workout; the harder you work, the better the results you get – guaranteed.

If you compare this with a 30-minute gentle bike ride or run, you would obviously still be burning calories, but not getting the same effect, as you will not have challenged the body hard enough to raise the EPOC.

I refer to this as the 4-minute miracle. This training can help melt fat super fast, can increase your aerobic capacity, anaerobic capacity, VO2 max, boost your resting metabolic rate, and can get you more toned and leaner.

HOW TO DO YOUR 4-MINUTE ROUTINE

Each routine has just two exercises, one of which you do for a total period of 20 seconds. This will be the high-intensity move. After you do this for exactly 20 seconds, you go straight into the second exercise, which will be low intensity. You do this one for 10 seconds. This is your recovery period when you get your breath back, and mentally prepare for the next intensity move.

NOTE

VO2 MAX IS A MEASURE OF THE MAXIMUM VOLUME OF OXYGEN THAT AN ATHLETE CAN USE. IT IS MEASURED IN MILLILITRES PER KILOGRAM OF BODY WEIGHT PER MINUTE (ML/KG/MIN).
IT IS THE INTENSITY OF A WORKOUT THAT GAINS YOU THE MAXIMUM RESULTS, NOT THE DURATION, SO LESS IS MORE.

You continue this cycle for a total of eight rounds making a total of four minutes – it's as simple as that.

As simple as it is, this an incredible workout. If you push yourself hard in the 20-second bursts, you can expect to see some pretty amazing results with your improved fitness and body shape.

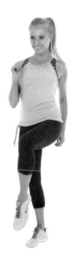

Level 1
Low-impact – ideal for beginners

Level 2
Moderate – for beginner to intermediate levels

Level 3
Hard – suits people who are reasonably fit

Level 4
Very hard and high-impact – for the very fit

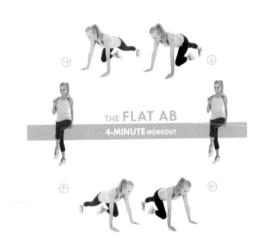

THE **FLAT AB**
4-MINUTE WORKOUT

I have put together a total of 10 different 4-minute workout variations. Some are more challenging than others so I have graded the routines for you.

HOW TO WARM UP, STRETCH AND COOL DOWN

While each workout is only four minutes, it is important to warm up and cool down to help prevent injuries and to stretch out the muscles you are using.

These are elements of a workout that often get ignored. However, they are important to help you perform better, and to help prevent injuries. So I urge you to warm up before you do any of the workouts and cool down afterwards.

WARM UP

For your 4-minute workouts, even though these are super short, it is still important to warm up. Consider spending a couple of minutes walking up and down the stairs, or perhaps do a brisk walk around the garden.

For the longer workouts, when you are heading outdoors to do your running or walking, it is a good idea to spend a couple of minutes walking at a moderate pace, and gradually build up speed so by the end of the two minutes, you are walking at a good brisk pace. This will help increase your core body temperature, and the motion of walking is a great way of lubricating your joints and muscles. This means by the time you are into the workout proper, your muscles are simply more pliable, making the exercise easier.

Bear in mind that on a very hot day your body temperature will naturally be higher, as opposed to a cold day when you may want to spend longer warming up. As a good rule of thumb, always ensure you feel warm before you start exercising.

COOL DOWN

Many people think that once they have finished exercising it's okay to just stop. This should be avoided. It is far better to slowly reduce the pace. So if you are back from a walk or run and if you have done your 4-minute workout, just march around the room for a minute or so to slowly bring your body back to its pre-exercise state.

In short, always make sure you warm up and cool down.

THE IMPORTANCE OF STRETCHING

Your warm-up stretches are an important part of your training, and also help keep you flexible and your body in alignment, so it is always good practice to do your stretches both before and after.

CALF STRETCH

Step back with one leg, and keep the heel down, with both feet pointing forwards. Rest your hands on the bent leg. Hold for 10 seconds.

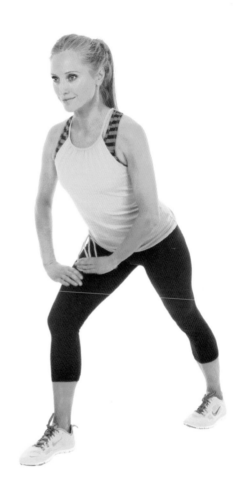

HAMSTRING STRETCH

Standing straight, bend one leg and extend the other out straight, with heel on the floor and toes pointing up. Place both hands on bent leg. Stick your bottom out to feel the stretch along the back of the straight leg. Hold for 20 seconds on each leg.

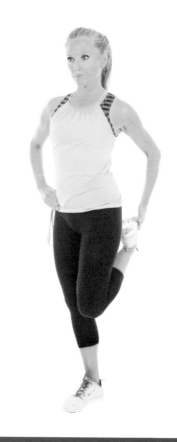

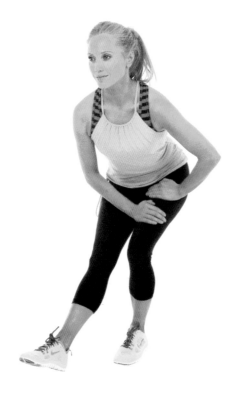

QUAD STRETCH

Stand with good posture, bend one leg behind you and gently hold the foot or sock of the bent leg. Push your hips forward to feel the stretch in the front of your thigh. Keep the supporting knee slightly bent. Hold for 10 seconds on each leg.

CHEST STRETCH

Stand with good posture, take your arms behind you, and lift your shoulders up and back to feel the chest stretch. Hold for 10 seconds.

BACK STRETCH

Stand with good posture, knees soft, and tummy pulled in. Take your arms in front of you and imagine you are hugging a big beach ball. Feel the stretch in your back. Hold for 10 seconds.

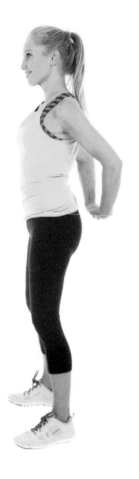

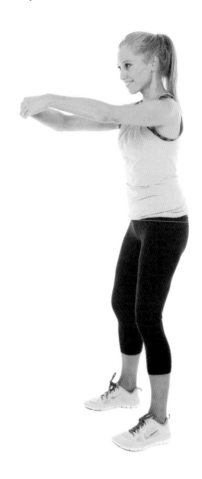

TRICEPS STRETCH

Stand with a strong, firm, straight back, knees slightly bent and tummy pulled in. Lift one arm up and bend it behind your head, aiming to get your hand between your shoulder blades. Hold for 10 seconds.

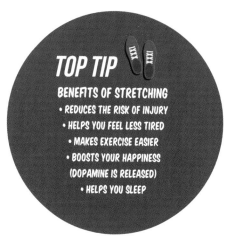

TOP TIP

BENEFITS OF STRETCHING
- REDUCES THE RISK OF INJURY
- HELPS YOU FEEL LESS TIRED
- MAKES EXERCISE EASIER
- BOOSTS YOUR HAPPINESS (DOPAMINE IS RELEASED)
- HELPS YOU SLEEP

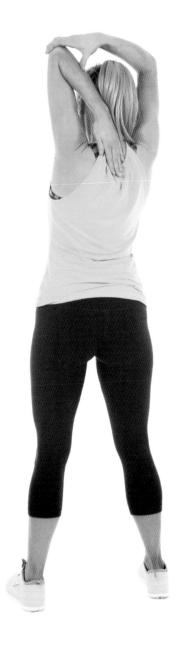

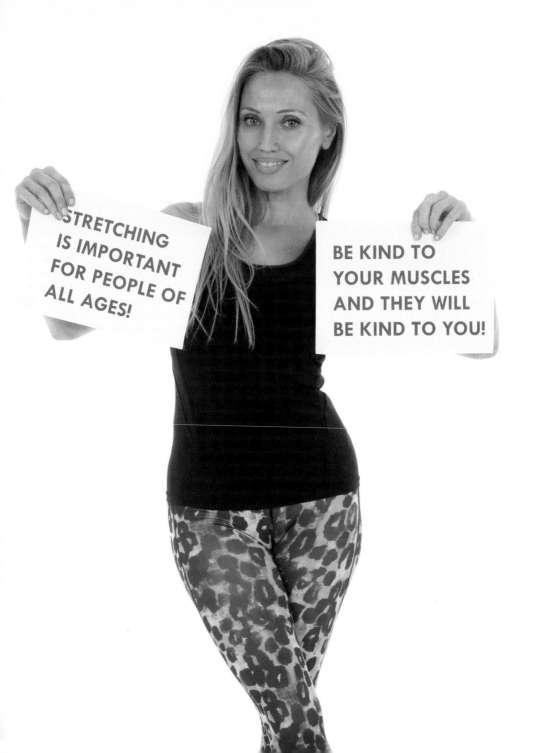

CHAPTER FIVE

4-MINUTE WORKOUTS

The workouts are listed in order from Level 1 to Level 4. Choose between easier and more difficult workouts over time for maximum benefit.

Find the right time for you to do your workouts. If you're an early morning person, this is a great time to do your 4-minute workouts – your body will be burning off those excess calories for the rest of the day. If you're not a morning person, don't force yourself to do your 4-minute workouts in the morning. Instead aim to squeeze them in at lunch time or late afternoon. Ultimately the best time to do your 4-minute routine is whenever it suits you best. Then make it a habit.

Playing music during your workout can help motivate you. Choose a tune that is upbeat and gets you in the mood to move. And as the workouts are just four minutes, you only need one song. Each day/week you might want change the tune to keep it interesting.

You'll need your stopwatch, your workout kit and a good pair of trainers.

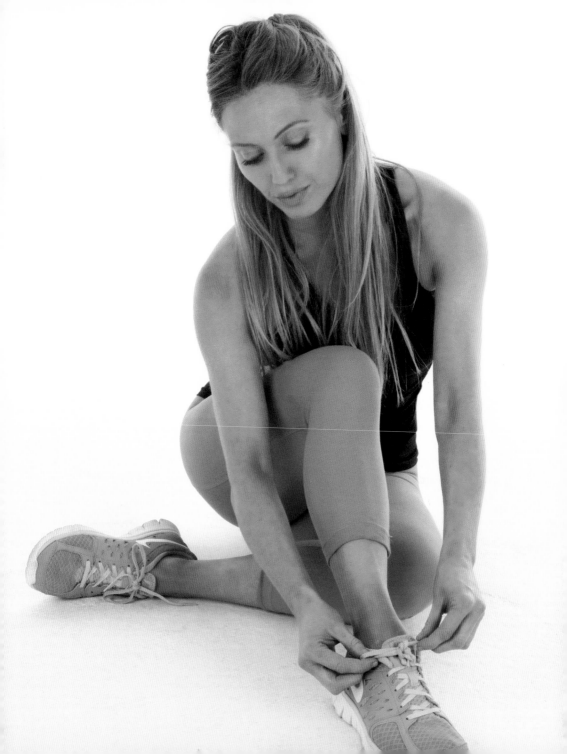

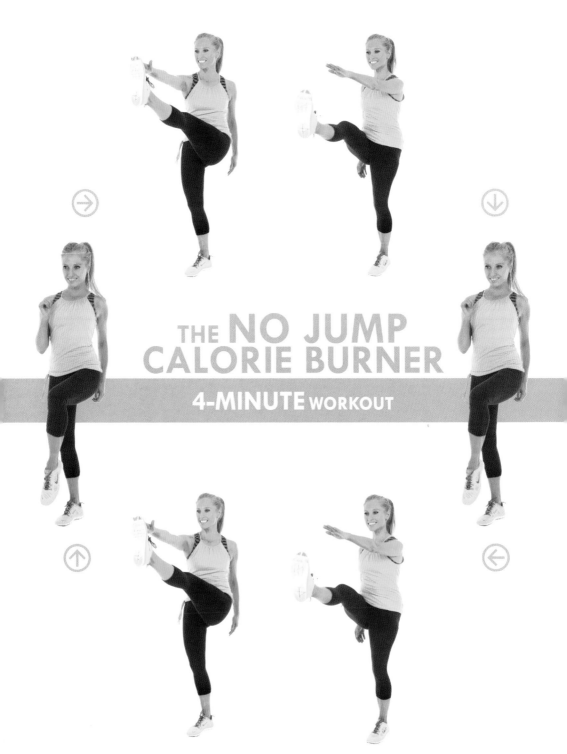

THE **NO JUMP**
CALORIE BURNER

4-MINUTE WORKOUT

NO JUMP CALORIE BURNER – LEVEL 1

This workout engages all your major muscles through a full range of movement, which makes this one a great calorie burner. This will help to tone your arms, bottom and legs. Make sure you complete your warm up before you start the workout, and perform your cool down at the end.

INTENSITY EXERCISE: LEG KICK

In an upright position, simply kick one leg straight out in front, and aim for your opposite hand to reach your foot. Then lower your leg and arm, and kick the other leg up reaching with the opposite hand.

Keep alternating this move for a total of 20 seconds, making sure you keep your back straight and your abdominals pulled in tight.

Follow this with the recovery exercise: Marching on the spot for 10 seconds.

Repeat these two exercises one after the other for a total of eight times, and that is your 4-minute workout done.

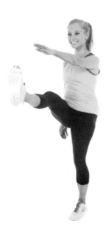
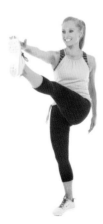

WONDER WAIST WORKOUT – LEVEL 1

This move is low-impact, and is great for toning into your waistline and helping to shape and sculpt your arms. This looks easy, but you would be amazed at how just using your arms can quickly crank up the intensity of the workout, and as we know, it is intensity that gets us results. Perform your warm up first and always complete your cool down at the end of the workout.

INTENSITY EXERCISE: WAIST PUNCH

Standing in a wide stance with your knees slightly bent and tummy muscles pulled in, simply punch your arms from side to side, keeping them at chest height and making sure you keep your hips still. Be sure to punch out wide, so you can feel it working in the sides of your waist. Do this for 20 seconds.

Follow this with the recovery exercise: Marching on the spot for 10 seconds.

Repeat these two exercises one after the other for a total of eight times, and that is your 4-minute workout done.

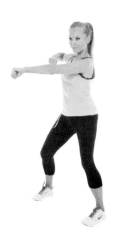 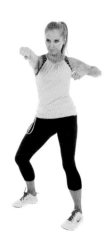

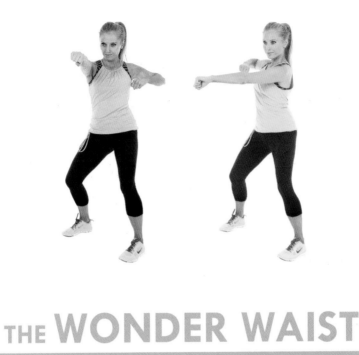

THE WONDER WAIST

4-MINUTE WORKOUT

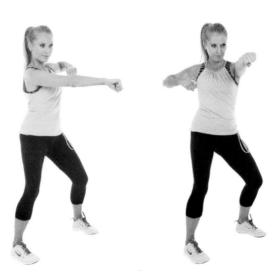

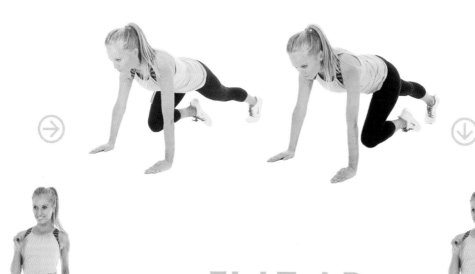

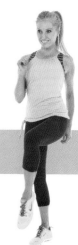

THE **FLAT AB**
4-MINUTE WORKOUT

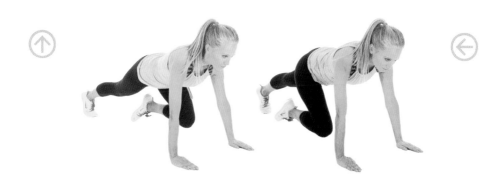

FLAT AB WORKOUT – LEVEL 2

This floor-based workout is not only a fat burner but also a great ab toning move, as you engage all the 3 muscle groups in your mid-section: your obliques, transverse abdominis, and rectus abdominis. So not only do we burn fat but we also are going to sculpt deep into those tummy muscles.

INTENSITY EXERCISE: AB TONING

Starting in a plank position, bring one knee in, aiming to get your thigh towards your chest. Hold, then jump leg back, and alternate to bring opposite knee in towards the chest. Throughout the move focus on keeping your abdominals pulled in tight. Do this for 20 seconds.

Follow this with the recovery exercise: Marching on the spot for 10 seconds.

Repeat these two exercises one after the other for a total of eight times, and that is your 4-minute workout done.

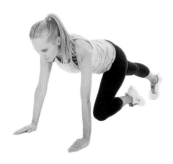 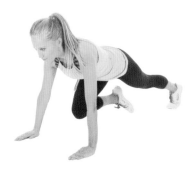

JOG-IT-OFF WORKOUT – LEVEL 2

This is as easy as it sounds. You literally just jog on the spot for 20 seconds. But the jogging will help increase your heart rate, and the faster and higher you get those knees up, the more calories you will be burning for the rest of the day. So if you want a simple move but powerful results, then this is a great workout to choose.

INTENSITY EXERCISE: JOGGING ON THE SPOT

Aim to get your knees high and pump through with your arms, keeping them bent at the elbows. Aim to land softly, and keep the tummy muscles pulled in tightly. Do this for 20 seconds.

Follow this with the recovery exercise: Marching on the spot for 10 seconds.

Repeat these two exercises one after the other for a total of 8 times, and that is your 4 minutes.

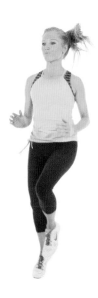

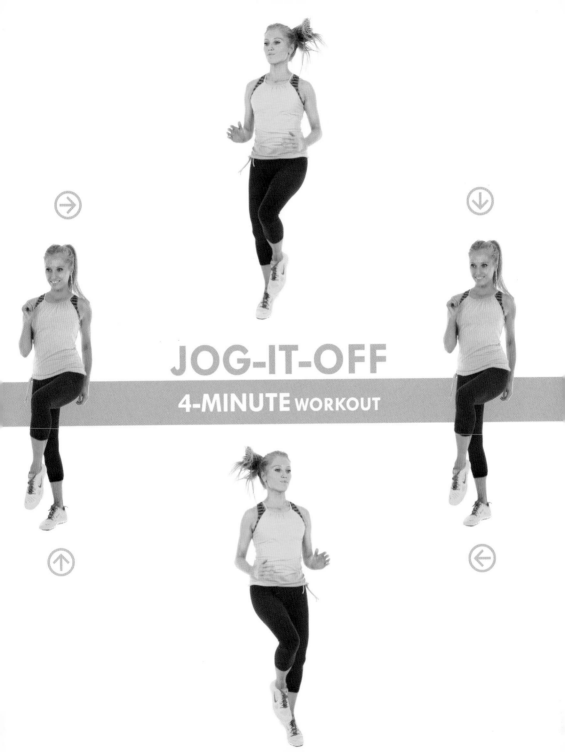

JOG-IT-OFF

4-MINUTE WORKOUT

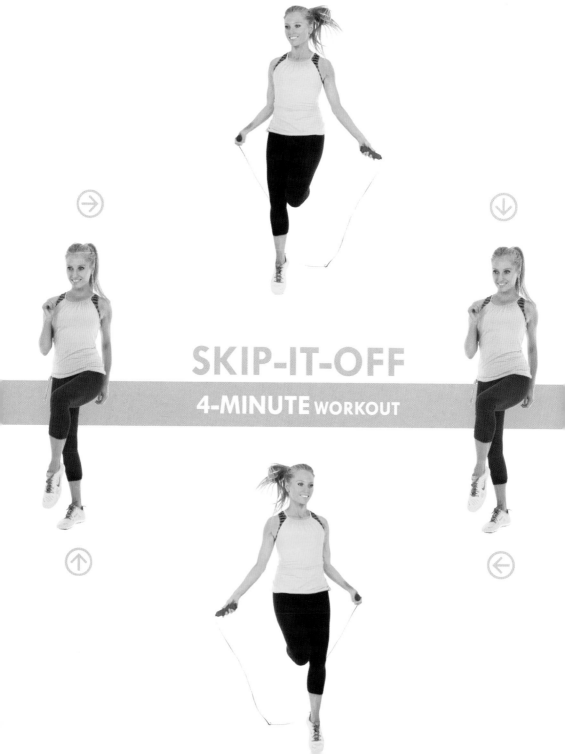

SKIP-IT-OFF

4-MINUTE WORKOUT

SKIP-IT-OFF WORKOUT – LEVEL 2

Skipping is a great way to shift fat and tone up. And don't be put off if you think you can't skip, as you can start without a skipping rope and simply mimic the skipping move, and within a few sessions you will be able to add that rope and find that skipping will become your thing. As always with any high impact move, try and focus on landing softly. Be sure to warm up first before you start the workout, and perform your cool down at the end.

INTENSITY EXERCISE: SKIPPING

With a skipping rope, aim to jump off the floor, giving the rope just enough space to slip under your feet. Only the balls of your feet should touch the floor. Keep your elbows bent, and aim to land softly. Do this for 20 seconds.

Follow this with the recovery exercise: Marching on the spot for 10 seconds.

Repeat these two exercises one after the other for a total of eight times, and that is your 4-minute workout done.

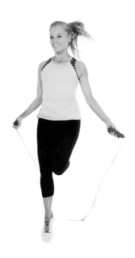

LOWER BODY WORKOUT – LEVEL 3

This workout targets your legs, bottom, hips, thighs, waist and abdominals. The benefit of this is that you are toning major muscle groups. These dynamic compound moves will supercharge your calorie burn. Make sure you complete your warm-up before you start the workout, and perform your cool down at the end.

INTENSITY EXERCISE: SKI SQUAT JUMP

Start in a squat position with knees bent and your arms extended out in front. Be sure that your knees are behind the line of your toes.

Jump high and land 180 degrees to the left in your deep squat position. Hold, then jump back to the right. Keep doing this for a total of 20 seconds.

Follow this with the recovery exercise: Marching on the spot for 10 seconds.

Repeat these two exercises one after the other for a total of eight times – that's your 4-minute workout done.

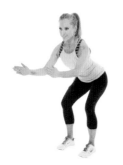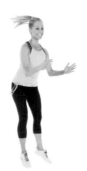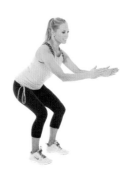

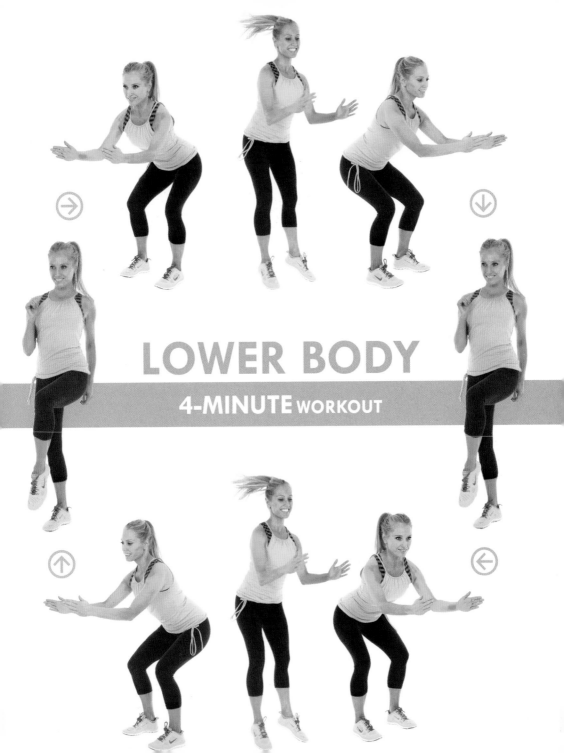

LOWER BODY
4-MINUTE WORKOUT

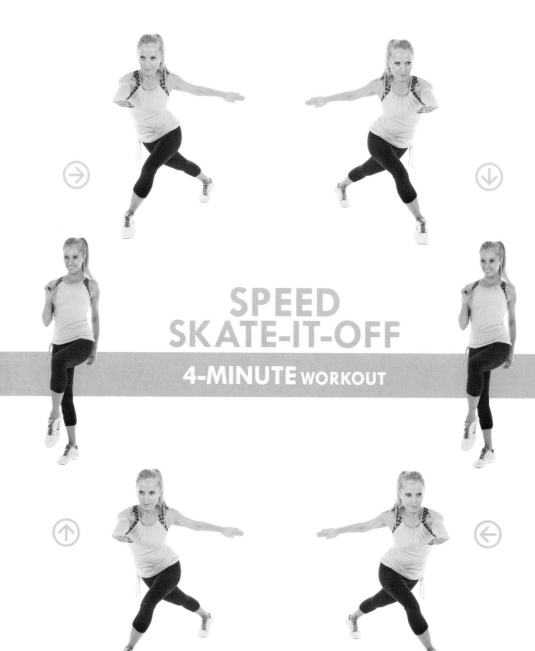

SPEED
SKATE-IT-OFF
4-MINUTE WORKOUT

SPEED SKATE-IT-OFF WORKOUT – LEVEL 3

This dynamic move, which is similar to that performed when speed skating, engages lots of muscles groups, and uses what is known as a lateral movement as you jump from side to side. This one is great for full body toning, and also helps to speed up that metabolism. Perform your warm up first, and don't forget to cool down when you finish.

INTENSITY EXERCISE: SPEED SKATER LUNGE

Aim to keep your hips square during this exercise. Place your right foot diagonally behind you, heel lifted. Lower into a lunge – don't let the front knee go past toes. Extend right arm across your body and your left arm out to the side. Now switch to the other side, adding a jump as you change from one leg to the other. (If you are a beginner, just step across.) Do this for 20 seconds.

Follow this with the recovery exercise: Marching on the spot for 10 seconds.

Repeat these two exercises one after the other for a total of eight times, and that is your 4-minute workout done.

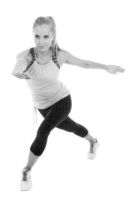 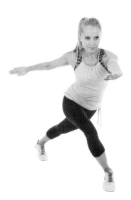

STAR SQUAT JUMP WORKOUT – LEVEL 3

This move works your arms and legs by extending arms and legs out to your sides as you jump to make a star shape. It's a great fat-melting move – the higher you jump and the lower you land, the more calories you burn.

INTENSITY EXERCISE: STAR SQUAT

Starting in a deep squat position, hold and then jump up as high as you can as you swing your arms and legs out wide. Land back to your deep squat position. Repeat for 20 seconds.

Follow this with the recovery exercise: Marching on the spot for 10 seconds.

Repeat these two exercises one after the other for a total of eight times, and that is your 4-minute workout done.

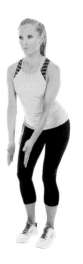 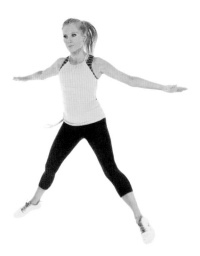

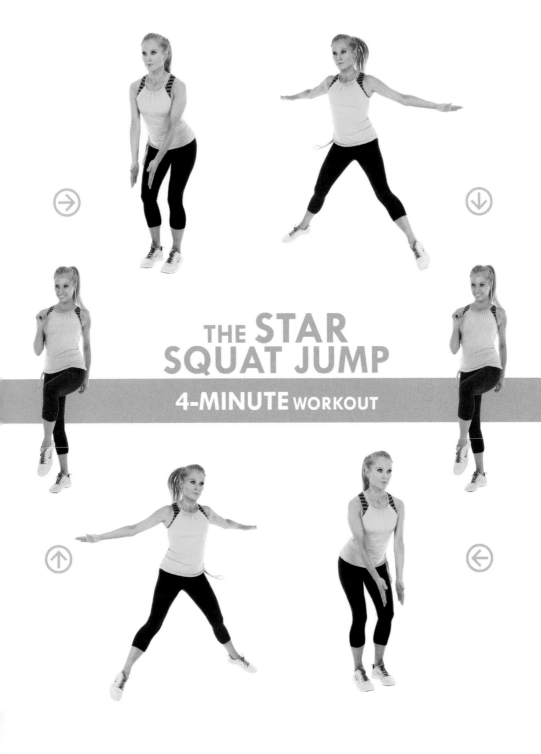

THE **STAR**
SQUAT JUMP
4-MINUTE WORKOUT

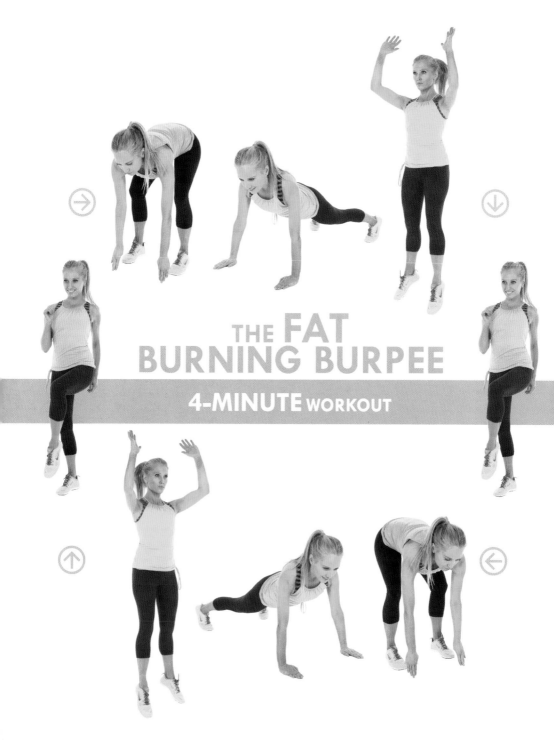

THE **FAT** BURNING BURPEE

4-MINUTE WORKOUT

FAT BURNING BURPEE WORKOUT – LEVEL 4

This one is tough – the famous burpee. Not only is this high impact, but also the range of the movement is from a very low plank position to a high jump, which engages nearly all muscle groups and makes this an excellent fat burner. Always be sure to complete your warm up first and then cool down at the end.

INTENSITY EXERCISE: FAT BURNING BURPEE

Start the exercise standing, then bend through the knees so your hands can touch the floor, then jump your feet out to a plank position. Hold, then jump your feet back in, and jump up high, aiming to land softly. Keep doing this for 20 seconds.

Follow this with the recovery exercise: Marching on the spot for 10 seconds.

Repeat these two exercises one after the other for a total of eight times, and that is your 4-minute workout done.

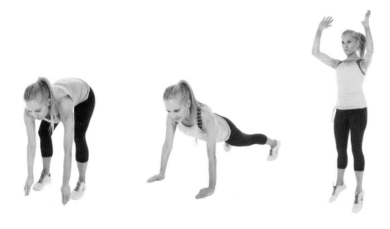

POWER JUMP WORKOUT – LEVEL 4

This workout is tough and involves a style of move known as plyometric – an explosive jump motion. The results of this workout are two-fold: your body will burn calories at a much higher rate, and you chisel and sculpt your body all over.

This is a hard workout and not recommended for beginners. Perform your warm up first and don't forget to cool down at the end.

INTENSITY EXERCISE: JUMPING

Starting in a slight squat position, with your hands by your knees, jump up high, aiming to tuck your knees in as tight as you can, then land back to your start position. Aim to do this for 20 seconds.

Follow this with the recovery exercise: Marching on the spot for 10 seconds.

Repeat these two exercises one after the other for a total of eight times, and that is your 4-minute workout done.

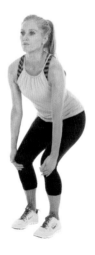 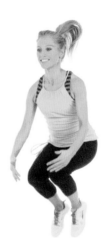

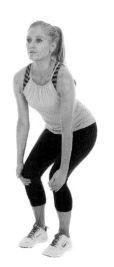
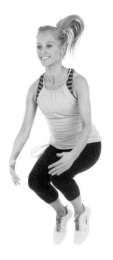

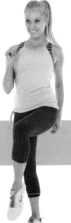

THE **POWER JUMP**
4-MINUTE WORKOUT

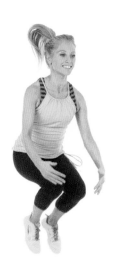
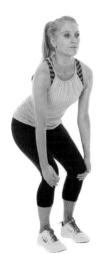

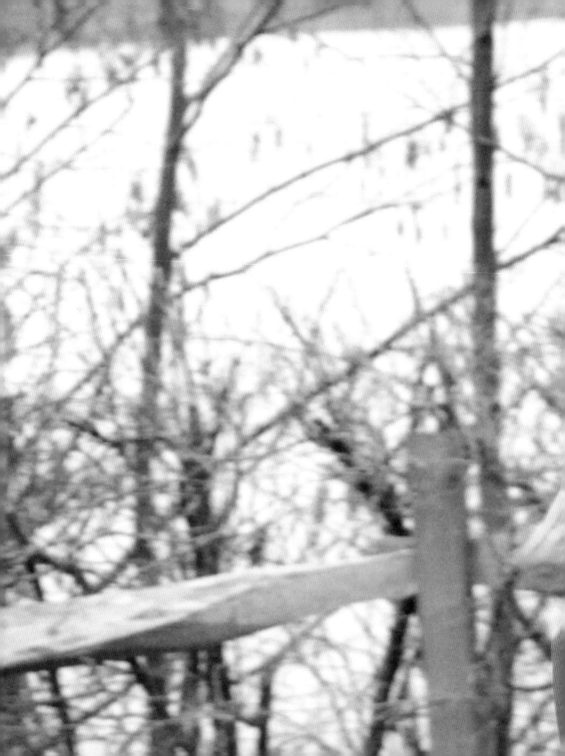

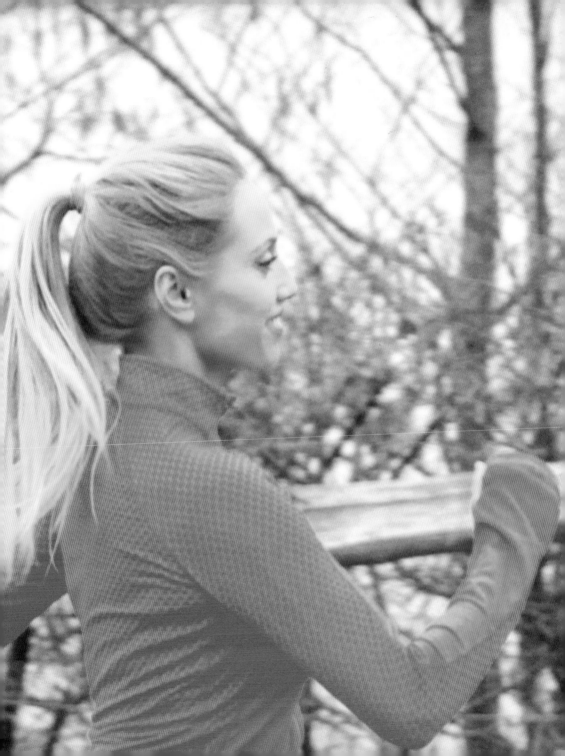

CHAPTER SIX

WALK/RUN EXERCISES

The fast 4-minute exercises are central to the program. You can supplement these with my 16-minute fat burning ab toning walk and the 21-minute fat burning interval run. Both will help tone your body, improve your fitness, strength and bone density.

Make sure you have some good-quality joggers – it's best to have your running shoes professionally fitted. And take water with you to stay hydrated.

If you don't like running, that's OK. Just do the 16-minute interval fat burning, ab toning walk.

Walking and running are great ways to keep fit and stay in shape. And they are exercises you can do with friends.

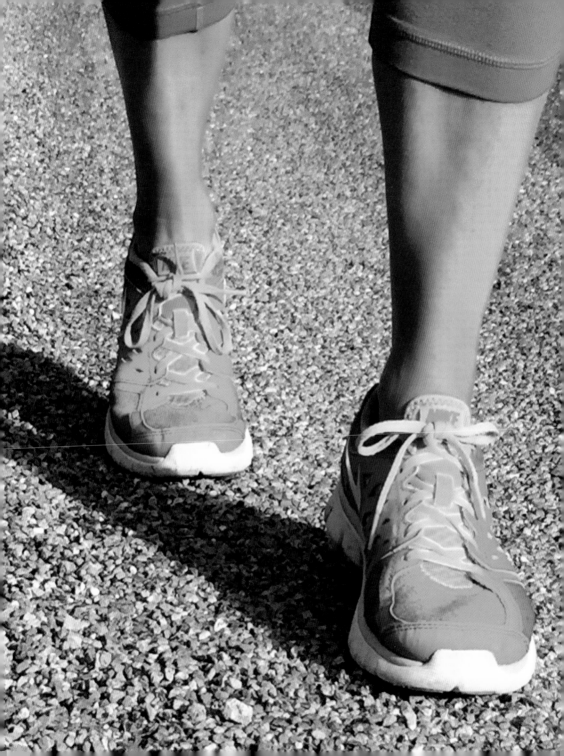

WALK IT OFF

Walking is one of the most natural exercises we can do and is a great way to burn excess body fat. Walking is something we all do so it can be easy to squeeze into a busy day. These days we can get somewhere faster by walking than perhaps driving and being stuck in traffic.

So there are two options you have: you can either aim to complete a certain amount of steps in one day by wearing a pedometer, as I mentioned in Chapter 1, or you can try my special fat burning walking workout.

The pedometer option will give you some goals to aim for. Start by wearing your pedometer on a normal day (without thinking about your goals) to see how many steps you clock up – you might be surprised as to how many. Then whatever your result is, aim to increase this by around one thousand steps each day.

Your ultimate goal is going to be between 7 and 10 thousand steps, at least three times a week. If you are already at this number, then simply keep up the good work.

THE BENEFITS OF WALKING

Walking is very good for us in so many ways.

- Helps to lower the risk of heart disease and diabetes, and reduce the risk of a stroke
- Helps to lower your cholesterol and blood pressure
- Helps lubricate your joints, keeping you supple and flexible
- Low-impact so it is ideal for every fitness level
- Helps to raise levels of feel-good hormones reducing anxiety and stress.
- Helps to keep your muscles active and lean
- Helps raise your metabolism which prevents your body storing excess fat
- Helps keeps your bones strong and will help prevent osteoporosis

As with all exercise, walking helps to slow the aging process, as it stimulates the Human Growth Hormone which is responsible for keeping us looking younger.

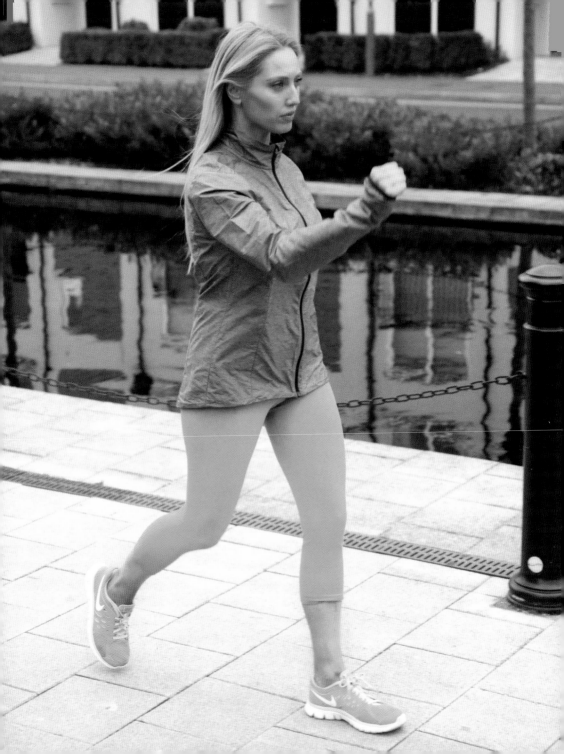

Your choice: you can either aim to build up your number of steps to 10 thousand steps at least three days a week, which is equivalent to a workout. Or you can follow my 16-minute fat burning, ab toning walking workout.

First, let's look at how to walk to maximise benefits.

HOW TO WALK WITH GOOD TECHNIQUE

- Keep good upright posture through your upper body. Visualise that you have to keep your shoulders stacked directly above your hips; this will help you to maintain that upright posture.
- Your arms should be bent at a 90-degree angle.
- Swing arms forward and back. It is important however not to swing the elbows higher than your shoulders.
- Always imagine you are walking along a straight line, this helps keep your joints in alignment.
- As you walk, push off with your toes, and concentrate on landing on your heel, rolling through the step, and pushing off again with your toes.
- Focus on keeping your pelvis and hips as relaxed as possible, so that you are able to walk freely with your legs, and engage a full range of movement.

It is always important to warm up before any exercise and this applies to my 16-Minute Fat Burning & Ab Toning Walk. For this I recommend that you simply spend a couple of minutes walking at a gentle pace.

At the end of the workout you should spend one minute cooling down by simply reducing the speed you are walking at until you come to a gradual halt, and finishing off with any of the cooling down stretches shown earlier in this book.

16-MINUTE FAT BURNING AND AB TONING WALK

Minutes 1 to 3	Simply walk at a brisk pace. Move your arms and maintain a good pace.
Minutes 4 to 5	Still walking at your brisk pace with good posture, pull your belly button in as tightly as you can towards your spine and maintain for a count of 10 seconds, then release for 10 seconds. Keep repeating this for one minute.
Minutes 6 to 7	Speed up and walk as fast as you can.
Minutes 8 to 10	Same as the first three minutes, walk at a brisk pace, move your arms and maintain a good pace
Minutes 11 to 12	Still walking at your brisk pace, pull your belly button in as tightly as you can towards your spine and maintain for a count of 10 seconds, then release for 10 seconds. Keep repeating this for one minute.
Minutes 13 to 14	Now up the speed of your walk and walk as fast as you can.
Minutes 15 to 16	Walk at a brisk pace, move your arms and maintain a good pace.

RUN IT OFF

Running has great benefits for keeping you in shape, keeping your heart and lungs healthy, and it supercharges your energy and decreases your stress levels. And this is exercise you can do anywhere, even during a lunch break.

One of the best benefits of running is that it helps to shed fat fast, particularly belly fat. The reason why running has such a quick effect on weight loss is that, on average, running for 15 minutes can burn up to 250 calories. This obviously varies for each individual, as we all burn calories at different rates, but this figure shows why running is called a **high-calorie burner** – together with walking and the 4-minute workouts.

When you run you engage nearly all your major muscles groups from your legs to your torso and your arms. You will start to notice your body firming up, in a number of ways.

One area you will notice quickly is your stomach, as running has a great impact on making your waist smaller and tummy flatter. This is due to the calorie burn and also the constant use of the oblique muscles that run down the side of the waist, as we engage these constantly when we are running. You then also get a lifted butt, as running tones up your gluteals, which are your bottom muscles, especially when you add slight inclines or even just the faster intervals, which will give your butt an extra lift.

HOW TO RUN WITH GOOD FORM

There is no such thing as the perfect running style, as everyone is different and has their own unique way of running. Next time you see runners on TV, look at how each runs differently; yet they are all still great runners. In saying that, the following tips will allow you to perfect your own running style and get the most out of every stride you take.

Your height, weight and body shape will determine the length of your natural running stride. Your running stride and how often you run will determine how fast you run. This, simply, is why we all run differently.

Let's have a look at the major body

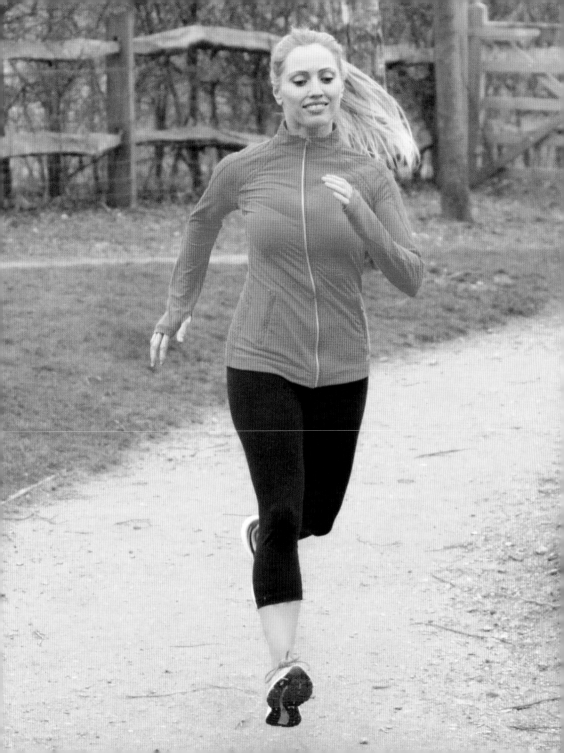

parts and how you can adjust your stance and position so that when you are running, you can focus on the right technique.

UPPER BODY

Keep your chest open, shoulders pulled back and down.

LEGS

The main power of your running comes from your legs. You naturally engage your legs from your core muscles. Imagine you are trying to pull your belly button in towards your spine, this helps keep your core in alignment.

ARMS

Focus on your lower arms below the elbow being bent at a 90-degree angle.

Keep your arms relaxed as you move, so they complement your natural running pace.

HANDS

It is very easy to clench your fists while you are running, but instead, focus on keeping your hands relaxed. Imagine that you are holding an eggshell between your thumb and forefinger without breaking it, so that your hands are still cupped without being clenched.

FEET

We are all individuals which means the way we land on our feet is different. There are two basic ways of landing: heel striker or toe striker.

If you are a heel striker, then you land on your heel of your front foot and then roll forward to push off from your toes.

If you are a toe striker, you land on your toes and push off from your heel. Whether you are heel or toe, just do what feels the most natural to you.

BEFORE YOU START

It is important to warm up and not just go straight into a run. Spend a couple of minutes walking, and gradually increase your walking speed so that towards the end of your warm up, you are walking at a good brisk pace. This will actually make running feel easier, as you will have warmed up all your muscles and lubricated your joints. This will help you to be more relaxed than if you are running when your body is cold. At the end of the run make sure you complete the cool down stretches listed under 'The importance of stretching' in Chapter 4.

21-MINUTE FAT BURNING INTERVAL RUN

2 Minutes	Run at a comfortable pace.
40 Seconds	Increase your speed to a fast run.
20 Seconds	Take this to a sprint (as fast as you can run).
Repeat this routine seven times.	

CHAPTER SEVEN

PLAN YOUR WEEK AHEAD

YOUR WEEKLY PLANNER

This is a great way to get organised for the week ahead, so select the two days you choose to fast. Select the meals you plan to eat and add to your planning showing each mealtime (and snacks if you want, to make up your calorie count of 500 for women, 600 for men). Then select a workout for each of your non-fasting, workout days.

You can find the example weekly planner and the weekly planner template on pages 154 and 155. Photocopy the template so that each week you can fill out your weekly diet and workout routine. Stick it on the fridge door to help keep you motivated and focused. Alternatively, visit my website to download the planner template: www.lwrfitness.com/personalised-fast-diet-plans/

Once you have attained your weight loss goal, consider a 1:6 ratio with only one fasting day a week.

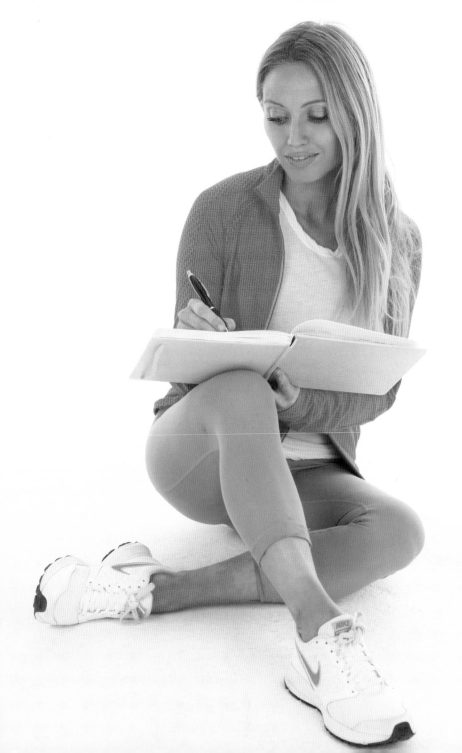

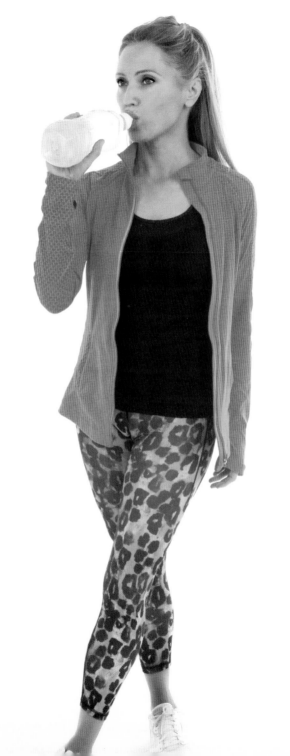

TOP 10 TIPS FOR YOUR FASTING DAYS

It's always a good idea to have a plan for your fasting days to help you to stick to the program. Here are some tips that can help you stay on track.

1. Make sure you choose a day that you are not rushing around.
2. Choose a day that you know you can grab an early night.
3. Make sure you have all the ingredients you need in stock.
4. Drink plenty of water.
5. If you get tempted to overindulge on your calories for the day, quickly grab the phone and distract yourself from that craving by phoning a friend.
6. Have a hot herbal tea, as this is only two calories, and often having something hot can satisfy any cravings.
7. Fill your car up with fuel the day before, to avoid being tempted by crisps or chocolate when you pay for your fuel.
8. Treat yourself to some magazines or a book to read to keep you busy and your mind occupied.
9. Distract yourself by having a day of de-cluttering a room or going through paperwork.
10. Especially for women, have this day also as a pampering day. Paint your nails, have a facial, visit a beauty salon and relax.

A FINAL WORD

What is important is to maintain a healthy weight. By this I mean not be overweight and equally as important, not to be underweight.

Once you have reached your healthy weight, it is easy to maintain if you stick with eating healthy, clean foods and by being active five times a week. Food is such a big part of our lives and should be enjoyed – it is not our enemy.

However, often busy lives and factors related to our lifestyles have not helped.

Do any of these factors ring a bell?
- We eat less homemade, fresh foods.
- Portion sizes have become larger.
- We often don't plan what we eat, so we eat on the run.

- We lead more sedentary lives – many people live on their computers or mobile devices.
- We can now do our grocery shopping online – at least visiting the supermarket meant walking up and down the aisles.

Despite these and other setbacks that prevent us from eating healthy food and living a healthy active life, it is possible to make the change that will have you feeling and looking great. You won't regret it and neither will your body and mind.

I leave you with one simple message: the best way to keep extra weight off is to eat fresh, homemade food and stay active.

Enjoy!
Lucy xox

KEEP IN TOUCH

I hope this book has shown you how simple the 5:2 diet can be with my easy-to-make healthy recipes. Together with the workouts, you'll get fast results.

I am a big fan of social media posting more recipes and workout options on my social media pages so do come and say hello and let me know how my fastest diet and workout program has worked for you. Share your success and any of your own recipes you have created. You can follow my 4-minute workouts in full on my YouTube channel.

Find me on:
Pinterest LWR Fitness
Facebook LWR Fitness
Instagram @lucywyndhamread
YouTube LWRFITNESS Channel
Twitter @lucywyndhamread
And for more information and my regularly posted blogs, visit:
www.lwrfitness.com

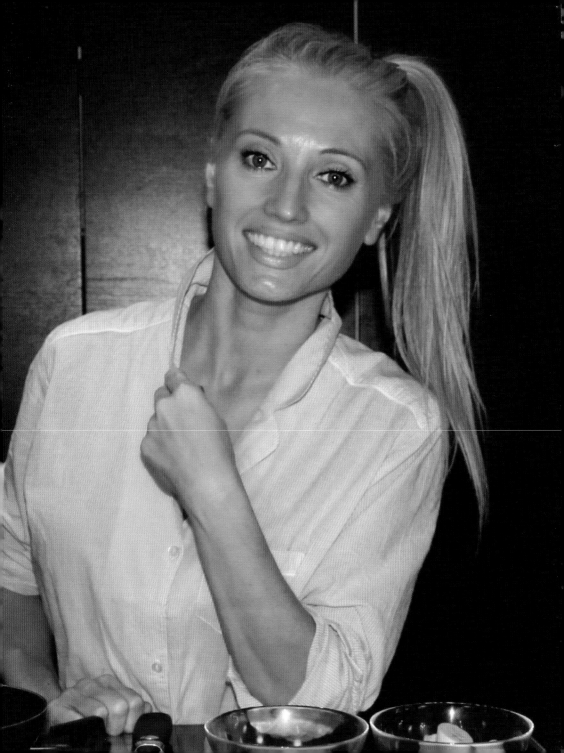

WEEKLY PLANNERS
EXAMPLE WEEKLY PLANNER

DAY	FASTING DAY /WORKOUT	DAILY MENU FOR FASTING/EXERCISE PLAN
MONDAY	Fasting Day	**Breakfast:** Mushroom and Spinach Cup Cake (50 calories) **Lunch:** Grilled Aubergine with Melted Chilli Haloumi (116 calories) **Dinner:** Fillet Steak on Carrot Noodles with Broccoli Florets (201 calories)
TUESDAY	Workout	4-minute Lower Body Workout
WEDNESDAY	Workout	4-minute Flat Abs Workout
THURSDAY**	Fasting Day	Breakfast: Egg and Bacon Muffin (191 calories) **Lunch:** Miso and Spring Vegetable Soup (97calories) **Dinner:** Chilli Con Carne (189 calories)
FRIDAY	Workout	4-minute Wonder Waist Workout
SATURDAY	Workout	16-minute Interval Fat Burning Ab Toning Walk
SUNDAY	Workout	4-minute Skip-it-off Workout

WEEKLY PLANNER

DAY	FASTING DAY /WORKOUT	DAILY MENU FOR FASTING/EXERCISE PLAN
MONDAY		
TUESDAY		
WEDNESDAY		
THURSDAY		
FRIDAY		
SATURDAY		
SUNDAY		

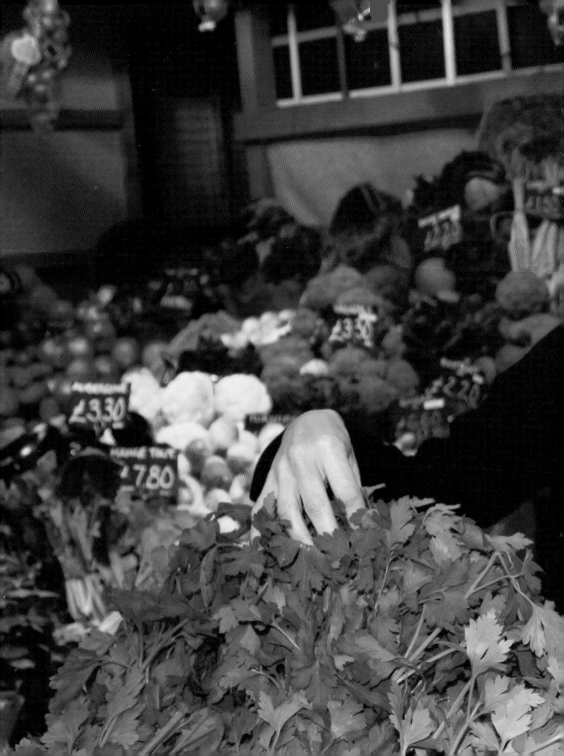

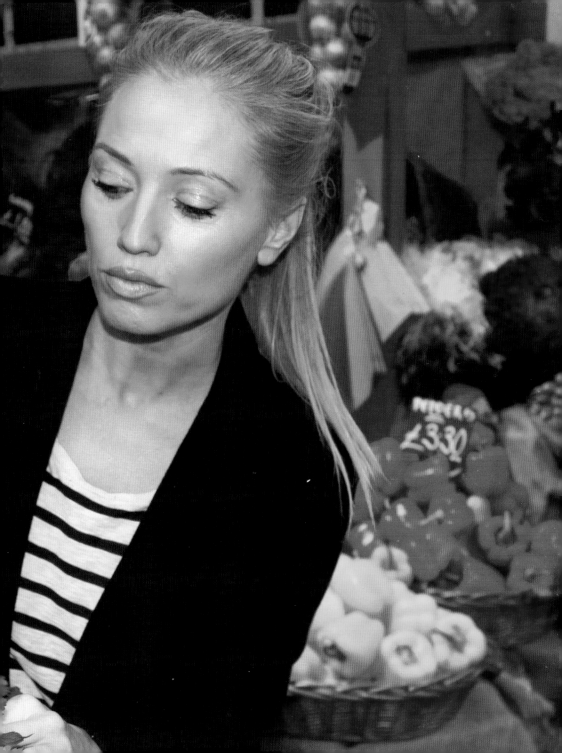

ACKNOWLEDGEMENTS

I would like to thank a few people that have been involved in the process of creating and writing this book. Firstly, I'd like to thank my wonderful family who have encouraged me and have been wonderful support. Thank you Keith for the huge task of proofreading my draft manuscript and Axl Stone for the exercise photos.

For your own personally devised Fast Diet plan and online one-to-one consultation, please visit www.lwrfitness.com/personalised-fast-diet-plans/

PHOTO CREDITS

Exercise photographs, by Axl Stone
Recipe images, © Lucy Wyndham-Read
Shutterstock for images in Top Tips and Notes
Susie Stevens (bold-type.com.au) for image page 100
Michael Lloyd for images pages 10, 31, 34, 153, 156

First published in 2015 by New Holland Publishers Pty Ltd
London • Sydney • Auckland

The Chandlery Unit 009 50 Westminster Bridge Road London SE1 7QY United Kingdom
1/66 Gibbes Street Chatswood NSW 2067 Australia
5/39 Woodside Ave Northcote, Auckland 0627 New Zealand

www.newhollandpublishers.com

A record of this book is held at the British Library and the National Library of Australia.

ISBN 9781742577159

Managing Director: Fiona Schultz
Publisher: Alan Whiticker
Project Editor: Susie Stevens
Designer: Andrew Quinlan
Proofreader: Jessica McNamara
Production Director: Olga Dementiev
Printer: Toppan Leefung Printing Limited

10 9 8 7 6 5 4 3 2 1

Disclaimer
Care has been taken with the calorie count of each recipe but these will vary and are approximate guides. Consult your doctor before starting a new diet or fitness routine. Please do not exercise if you feel unwell or have an injury. This diet is not recommended for children, pregnant women or those who are under weight.

Keep up with New Holland Publishers on Facebook
www.facebook.com/NewHollandPublishers